LOST
MEMORIES

Lost Memories

Melinda Fengel, RN, BSN

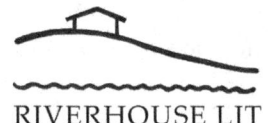

RIVERHOUSE LIT

Riverhouse Lit

Dewey, AZ 86327

Dewey, AZ 86327

Cover art by Donna Casey

Edited by Yoly Fivas

Interior type styles: Bookman Old Style, Tahoma

Note from the Editor

This book addresses the use of gender-related pronouns with an extended style of using male (his), female (her), or singular "they" with a hope that, in the future, linguists quell the muddy waters with a definitive number and gender-neutral structure.

Important Note

The information presented in this book is an expression of the author's experiences and intended for informational and educational purposes only, and not as a medical instructional manual This book does not replace professional treatment, and while it offers experiences and wisdom gained by the author, the author in no way is offering medical advice or directives. If you are seeking a medical opinion for yourself or your loved one, you are encouraged to see a doctor or other qualified health-care professional to make informed and balanced choices.

Anecdotes from the author's life, although based upon real incidents, contain situations where the names have been changed to protect family members, and may be composites.

ISBN-13: 978-1478134268
ISBN-10: 1478134267

Dedication

To my friend and editor, Yoly Fivas, without whom
this book would not have been possible!

To my sister, Karin, whom I love and who gave me my
education.

Contents

FOREWORD..1

Chapter One..7
    IN THE BEGINNING

Chapter Two...14
    THE REALITY OF DEMENTIA

Chapter Three..17
    DIFFICULT DAYS

Chapter Four..21
    DEMENTIA

Chapter Five...29
    TRANSITIONS

Chapter Six..32
    KINDS OF DEMENTIA - MCI

Chapter Seven...34
    KINDS OF DEMENTIA – TREATABLE ISSUES

Chapter Eight...39
    KINDS OF DEMENTIA – ALZHEIMER'S

Chapter Nine...47
    KINDS OF DEMENTIA – LEWY BODY

Chapter Ten...51
    FRONTOTEMPORAL, PICKS AND PROGRESSIVE APHASIA

Chapter Eleven..55
    PARKINSON'S AND HUNTINGTON'S DISEASES

Chapter Twelve..58
    KINDS OF DEMENTIA – KORSAKOFF'S SYNDROME

Chapter Thirteen..62
    VASCULAR DEMENTIA

Chapter Fourteen...65
    STAGES OF DEMENTIA

Chapter Fifteen..70
    A PSYCHIATRIST'S STORY

Chapter Sixteen...74
    DRUGS

Chapter Seventeen...80
    BEHAVIORS

Contents

Chapter Eighteen...85
    LEGAL ISSUES

Chapter Nineteen..91
    LIVING YOUR OWN LIFE: JUNE'S STORY

Chapter Twenty..99
    DRESSING

Chapter Twenty-one..103
    EATING

Chapter Twenty-two..107
    TIME TRAVELERS: TOM'S STORY

Chapter Twenty-three..112
    GROOMING

Chapter Twenty-four...116
    FINGERNAILS

Chapter Twenty-five...120
    TOENAIL FUNGUS

Chapter Twenty-six..123
    TEETH

Chapter Twenty-seven..127
    PHONE SERVICE: LOUIS' STORY

Chapter Twenty-eight..131
    SKIN INTEGRITY

Chapter Twenty-nine...136
    HALLUCINATIONS: GRACE'S STORY

Chapter Thirty..144
    INCONTINENCE

Chapter Thirty-one..150
    BACTERIA

Chapter Thirty-two..153
    CHANGING ROLES: SARA'S STORY

Chapter Thirty-three..160
    WALKING AND FALLS

Chapter Thirty-four...163
    WEIGHT AND DIABETES

Chapter Thirty-five...167
    TRAVELING

Contents

Chapter Thirty-six..171
    PETS: BOB'S STORY

Chapter Thirty-seven..174
    DREAM STATE

Chapter Thirty-eight...178
    "I WANT TO GO HOME"...

Chapter Thirty-nine..183
    KEEPING A LOVED ONE AT HOME

Chapter Forty...189
    TOOLS THAT HELP

Chapter Forty-one...194
    MASSAGE, AROMA, MUSIC, ART, EXERCISE, PET,
    AND REMINISCENCE THERAPIES

Chapter Forty-two...199
    OCCUPATIONAL THERAPY AND ADULT DAY CARE

Chapter Forty-three...202
    SURGERY

Chapter Forty-four..205
    THEORY OF PERSONALITY

Chapter Forty-five..209
    TAKE CARE OF YOURSELF

Chapter Forty-six...213
    WHAT TO BRING ALONG

Chapter Forty-seven..218
    WHEN IS A NURSING HOME APPROPRIATE?

Chapter Forty-eight..221
    DEATH

Chapter Forty-nine...227
    LIVING WITH DEMENTIA

About the Author...ccxxix

Appendix A..ccxxxi
    BOOKS AND DISCS

Appendix B...ccxxxiii
    LIST OF WEB SITES

FOREWORD

As a nurse, I wanted to write a book on dementia for a couple of reasons, the first of which is why I became involved in medicine. Medicine addresses itself to the *problem* the person has and the treatment of that illness. Nursing addresses itself to the *person* with the problem, and further, the *family* of which that person is a member. There is a saying in nursing that goes, "If one family member is sick, the entire family is ill." The whole family group no longer reacts to the ill member in the way they did before he or she became sick. Everyone in the family group must redefine their roles and interactions.

Secondly, there is a plethora of information available, and most of it is overwhelming. Who has the presence of mind to sift through all the information and take what applies only to them? I wanted to help by writing a concise, easy to read, and interesting book about the hardest job in the world: going through the disease process, with a whole skin.

Dementia is a blanket term that covers a myriad of illnesses. There are treatable dementias such as B-12 deficiency, hypothyroidism, drug interactions, or normal pressure hydrocephalus, which if caught early enough, can be reversed. These diseases can mimic the early stages of Alzheimer's, with shuffling gait, slowed or repetitive responses, or even hallucinations. Because symptoms can be confusing, I recommend that a person with any signs goes to his or her physician. Tests can be done to determine the cause of those symptoms, and potentially treatment can be recommended.

Denial is probably the biggest contributor to late diagnosis. No one wants to believe that the person they have loved, and have had a relationship with over many years, is slipping. Frequently a spouse or supporter will be in the habit of covering for his or her significant other—feeling obligated to do so. After all, supporters commit to caring for their spouses, for better or worse. The problem is that they do it well beyond the time it is beneficial and frequently make themselves sick in the process.

I had a patient, Bill, who had collapsed and was hospitalized with inadequate heart perfusion. He had been trying to take care of his wife (a former nurse) who had been diagnosed with Alzheimer's. He told me that he loved her to distraction and could not believe that this awful disease was taking her away from him. She had degenerated to the stage where she wandered constantly. This meant that no matter where she was, she walked continuously, but in no particular direction. Unable to focus on a task or item, she would wander into rooms wherever she was. If confronted with a blank wall, she might stay there, neither turning right nor left, and be unable to get out of the room, but continually moving her feet. He became completely responsible for her care; she could no longer dress herself or bathe. As she became less and less capable of taking care of herself, his physical administration of her bodily needs took the place of their former sex life, which had been complete and wonderful. His care of her became their intimacy, and he was reluctant to let go of this function. His fear was that he would lose her all over again. Just the thought of it increased his anxiety.

What had landed him in the hospital was trying to keep up with her wandering, which took place at all hours of the day and night. Her interrupted sleep pattern did not appear to affect her negatively, but he still needed his rest.

After much conversation with both the doctor and me, he agreed that her care was not a one-person job, and he acquiesced. He needed help. Bill secured for her a place in an expensive care home, catering to Alzheimer's patients.

The next time I saw Bill he was again admitted to the hospital for exhaustion. Although he had placed his wife in a really nice home, she cried frequently, and continuously said, "I want to go home." Thinking he could fulfill her request, he would take her out every weekend and bring her to the home they had shared for over sixty years. At first this appeared to placate her, although she continued her wandering. In a matter of weeks, he came to realize that she could no longer recognize him, their children, or the home in which she had spent all her adult life. She continued to cry, "I want to go home...I want to go home." This broke his heart, and the strain was more than he could bear. He finally realized what his kids had been saying all along. An Alzheimer's patient saying "I want to go home" is not due to a memory of a place to which they wish to return. It is a simple request to have his or her life back.

Hope is defined by the dictionary as a desire that holds the expectation of fulfillment. That is, we expect that our wishes will come true. In most instances when people become ill, we who love them have the hope that, with time and treatment, they will improve. In the case of someone with the diagnosis of Alzheimer's, that is not possible. Hope becomes the enemy. There can be no expectation of a person's improvement.

Family members sometimes feel that their loved one will get better if placed in a facility that is dedicated to the treatment of Alzheimer's patients. While this is the best place for someone with the disease, the person will continue to decline. That is not why such places exist. They exist because it takes special training to care for an Alzheimer's patient.

In order to give someone with this awful disease the best care possible, the nurses and caregivers need to understand the disease—what happens to the brain and body—so that the care they provide enhances the person's life experience, and does not make more problems than it solves. For instance, approaching someone with this disease incorrectly can startle them. They need to be approached quietly, from the front and spoken to softly. This knowledge requires training. Although anyone can be trained, someone who lacks the compassion for the job will not last.

That is not to say that an individual cannot enjoy who their loved one is becoming. Frequently, as the facade of social veneer falls away, people with Alzheimer's can be delightful, and enjoy things they formerly were unable to enjoy when the veneer was in place.

I wrote this book with the sincere hope that people assisting persons with this dreadful disease can make the compassionate decisions necessary to take care of themselves, as well as their loved ones.

Chapter One

IN THE BEGINNING

The first thing you may notice is that your loved one is asking the same question over and over again, one that you answered only a few moments ago. She may become lost in a familiar area—not knowing where she is or how to get home. If you have witnessed several of these "mistakes," it is time to talk to your loved one's primary care physician and to talk with the rest of your family. It is also not a bad idea to talk to the person who is making the mistakes. If together you can make a plan, all that follows will be easier—not without pain and perhaps fear—but easier and perhaps more smoothly.

Generally speaking, your loved one knows that something is changing. He or she is confused, frightened, and often in denial. If the person knows you have their best interests at heart, s/he has a better chance of facing the illness, secure in the knowledge that you, the rest of the family, and physician are willing to address this illness together, do what is best to protect her, and move forward as a group.

Unfortunately there are personalities that refuse to acknowledge what is happening. They will argue, fight, and generally deny that they have changed in any way. If this happens, professional assistance can help in order to get the person the care they need.

In this day and age, with television, the internet, and all the other forms of media bombarding us about all the things that can go wrong, it is difficult to believe that anyone having an extensive memory problem would not know something was amiss. However, fear and denial play a big part in an elderly person's pretending that there is no problem. If there is a spouse, he or she may have learned to compensate for the affected person and feel an obligation to continue the charade as a matter of loyalty.

Individuals often do not want to admit that they have a problem, but if the problem is interfering with day-to-day life, it needs to be acknowledged. In order to face it head on, improve symptoms, or even just slow the progression of the illness, early diagnosis is the key. Until one has a diagnosis, the person with the illness is floundering in the dark. It may be that there is a simple, physical problem that can be corrected, but may be exacerbated by ignoring the symptoms. Even though there is an understandable place for denial in the process, individuals do better when they know what they are dealing with.

Frequently people with a problem want to ignore it, hoping it will go away or that it is just temporary, but the reality is that *something is wrong*. The best way to assess the issue is a visit to your loved one's primary care physician who can take the necessary tests to eliminate a reversible physical condition. Problems like B-12 deficiency, hypothyroidism, drug interactions or depression can exhibit symptoms similar to those of early dementia. Blood tests, a Mini-mental Exam, and possibly an MRI (to rule out a stroke or tumors), may be necessary and these can only be performed with a physician's order. Occasionally, a primary care physician may not feel qualified to make a diagnosis of dementia, and in that case you can request a referral to a neuropsychologist or psychiatrist, depending on the complexity of the symptoms.

Losing car keys, or forgetting which row the car was parked in at the mall, is common. It really tells more about the of distraction, anxiety, or the level of complication in a person's life at that moment, than it does a serious problem.

There are signs and symptoms that may indicate the need for a medical evaluation: a new level of forgetfulness, difficulty understanding spoken or written words, ongoing difficulty with word retrieval, not knowing common facts, withdrawal, depression, exhibiting suspicion, anxiety, insomnia, fearfulness, hallucinations, agitation without reason, and purposeless wandering. There are other indicators like driving difficulty, inappropriate handling of finances, and neglect in self care, but these are often seen slightly later in the process and hopefully have been addressed before they can become a problem.

There is some question about whether or not it is important to have your loved one formally diagnosed with a particular type of dementia or even if it can be accurately done—it can be in some cases—but many forms of dementia are diagnosed by a process of elimination. Most importantly, diagnosis can lead to help. A point of argument says that if it is an early dementia with signs and symptoms showing up between the ages of sixty and seventy or earlier, diagnosis will have benefits in some areas, such as what to expect, how long the typical course of illness will be (no one can tell exactly), and any symptoms particular to that type of dementia. Families can pre-plan for care and look at finances. With certain types of dementia there are drugs that can slow the disease process, allowing individuals and their families more time together. The harsh reality is that someone with dementia will need escalating forms of help until the end of life.

Beyond getting the loved one help, it is most important to ensure safety. Driving a car can be dangerous even if someone is fully aware. It can be more dangerous if someone is upset or depressed, and much more dangerous if she is in the beginning stages of dementia. Some states like Florida, with a large retired population, will take a report at their license bureau and send an investigator to see if the person mentioned in the report is capable of driving. Other states may give people licenses if they are alive and can walk into the licensing office. The benefit of having the state decide is the level of objectivity.

Frequently people feel they are capable of driving when they are not, particularly men and anyone who has been driving a long time, or they may even feel that they have no alternative. A person's personal physician can be of tremendous help in this area, especially if you can speak with him or her ahead of time to apprise them of the situation. They can give your loved one an exam and explain, if necessary, it is no longer safe to drive. The person getting the news will not like it any better coming from the doctor, but may be more accepting of a medical decision.

The other big area of danger is cooking. Forgetting to turn off the stove, or misusing the microwave, is a common problem. You need to ask yourself, "Do I want to see the house burn down to preserve someone's dignity?" Unplug the stove and microwave. There are alternatives—one can get meals on wheels, someone to come in to cook a big meal at least once per day. Remember that older folks don't eat as much volume or as frequently as a middle-aged person does. It is also healthier for older adults to eat a bigger meal at noon and a lighter one in the evening as their digestive systems work more slowly.

If you believe your parent is becoming forgetful, there is an at-home test you can try. Please remember that this was discovered in only one small study and is not definitive for dementia (an M.D. performing a Mini-mental Exam will be more accurate). The results of this home test do not apply to anything but Alzheimer's. The study was done by the New York State Psychiatric Institute, which found that people with Alzheimer's disease, the most common form of dementia, were unable to identify certain odors. Smell, it appears, can be an early predictor of approaching difficulties. A list of odors people with Alzheimer's have difficulty or cannot identify are strawberry, smoke, soap, menthol, clove, pineapple, lilac, lemon and leather.

If you have questions about the status of a loved one's behavior, memory, or if they are declining, a physician is the appropriate person to ask.

Chapter Two

THE REALITY OF DEMENTIA

The following story illustrates what can happen when individuals have dementia, even if a friendship occurs over time.

There were two couples who had been friends since their children were small and they lived in the same neighborhood. They moved into a luxury retirement community and had apartments near one another. Because they were so close, as their need for physical help increased, both couples moved into the same assisted living community.

Jen, with her blond hair—augmented by the bottle—and good figure was a lady with a lot of panache. Tom, with his distinguished white hair and goatee, had quiet manners. They were in bridge club with Ben and Betty, and were all striving to win the award for Best Bridge Couple. Ben had been a concert violinist and professor, and they had all frequently attended music recitals together.

Ben was a small, quiet man who loved classical music. He continued to study violin into his 60's, even though he was considered one of the best in the country. Betty was small like Ben, but with a loud voice and a brash manner honed while living in New York.

Unfortunately, months after moving into the new community, Ben suddenly died of a heart attack, and about a year later, Jen died of diabetes. As both their respective spouses were gone, Tom and Betty did not want to "rattle around" alone in big apartments, so they choose to move into studio apartments next door to one another. Because of their shared grief, Tom and Betty grew very close. And also, Betty needed Tom's help.

Betty had been diagnosed at stage three Alzheimer's, needed a walker due to hip arthritis, and had severe macular degeneration. Betty had a much harder time getting around than Tom, who was quite spry for his age, which was eighty-five. Their attachment exceeded being just good friends; she relied on him both physically and emotionally. For his part, Tom showed endless patience for Betty, escorting her down stairs via the elevator for every meal, and to many social activities.

Betty was not included in playing cards with friends because of her lack of vision and advanced dementia, but she would sit silently next to Tom while he played.

One day while sitting in the lobby chatting as they waited for the dining room doors to open for dinner, Betty suddenly paused, patted Tom on the knee and said, "What do I call you again, honey?"

The point of this story is both funny and sad, but as Betty's daughter said when I told her the story, "if you did not laugh at the funny things they say and do, you would cry all the time!"

Chapter Three

DIFFICULT DAYS

The most difficult days are in the beginning, when the person affected knows that something is not "right" with their thought processes, or at least something is not the same. Everyone who has dementia will progress to a point where they do not know what is happening, but in the early days, they are usually scared.

No one can give a family advice about how best to deal with the situations that arise. What I can tell you is, trust your instincts. The family actually knows their loved one best and knows inherently, the most sound approach to use. After all, family members have been dealing with the afflicted individual for years. What some members may require are practical suggestions and someone to help get all the other family members on track. It may be good to remember that while some familial relationships with the person in question may be excellent, there may be a family member who is in denial. Moreover, one or more of the family members may have a difficult or non-existent relationship with the person who is exhibiting symptoms. They may live further away and feel guilty about not participating in the family dynamics. Problems chiefly arise when the family is divided, or when one person is taking care of the loved one and the other family members either do no want to get involved, or are too busy with their own lives. Everyone needs to be on the same page. Denial can be lethal, both to the person who has the illness and to the relationships with the rest of the family. To help avoid this and other problems, the following is recommended:

1) Have a family meeting, make a flexible plan, and keep those lines of communication open. Let everyone participate to their capacity.

2) Consult with the person's primary care physician and get his/her help in talking to the person about safety measures (not driving), etc.

3) Get the loved one tested with a Mini-mental Exam (see later chapters for specifics), as well as any other kinds of tests the physician may recommend, in response to exhibited symptoms.

4) Talk to other people with the same problems. There are many support groups available. The Alzheimer's Society puts on all sorts of programs to educate families and caregivers. Talking to other people who are going through the same things can only help.

5) Ensure caregivers in the home understand the illness. This drill is not just about taking care of a normal elderly person.

6) Keep in your mind that there will come a time when the family will need to make decisions for the person—the person will become incapable. Take steps now to ensure that the transfer of personal decision making is smooth.

Remember to make goals for your loved one. Most people want the following:

1) Maintain quality of life. Stimulation that the person enjoys and is appropriate for them.

2) Provide as much independence as possible for as long as possible, within safety guidelines.

3) Supply first-class care to avoid things like skin breakdown, or any other problems arising from a lack of care.

No one wants their parent or other loved one to have this disease. It is not easy, but like most things in life, it can be managed with forethought and planning. It may even allow you to see a side of your loved one that you never knew existed.

Chapter Four

DEMENTIA

Dementia refers to a decline in cognitive functioning. There are several types of dementia with very different symptoms, but in all types, there is a decline in a person's ability to function and govern activities of daily living.

When I began subject research to write this book on dementia, I quickly realized that it would be impossible to compose a single book incorporating all the available information for this extensive topic. Beyond the overwhelming quantity of information, a great deal of available material is repetitive and relayed in a confusing manner. Some of the information applies to just one or two forms of dementia and would not relate to many people's experiences. So, what I have tried to do is take the most common information and coalesce this into a useable form, with many references for those individuals who wish to research on their own. By extending their research, they may uncover facts relevant or important to a particular situation. One of my primary goals is to empower individuals who have loved ones with dementia. Research, education, and choices made from a place of what is best for each individual's family are crucially important as one navigates this most difficult of situations.

Part of the problem is that denial works. No one in their right mind wants someone they love, or are even related to, to have this disease. Denial, as defined by the study of psychology, is the unconscious attempt to resolve an emotional conflict, and in the process allay the concomitant anxiety. No one wants to believe that their mother or father's functional level is changing. No one wants to admit that the person they love has begun a long, slow, slide into darkness, and that statement is even more true if the relationship between parent and child or remains unresolved. The down side of denial is that it keeps the person who is failing in limbo, without the help they really can get and desperately need.

There is help. Not a cure, but help and the first thing a family needs to do is find out as much as they possibly can from all available resources. As in any other venture, the trick is separating the reality from fiction. There is a plethora of knowledge available and one must compile it into a usable, relevant form from which decisions can be made. The old adage of "...if you read about an offer that seems to good to be true, it probably is..." goes for medications as well.

There is a good deal of experimentation and real research on the topic to investigate. One can sign up a parent for a study, but there is no guarantee that your loved one will get better, that the drug will work on a particular individual as it is designed to do, or even that your loved one will receive the drug being studied. In a double-blind study (which most legitimate studies are), the participants are split into two groups, and even many of the participating physicians don't know which members actually receive the drug being studied until after the study has been completed. That may mean Mom or Dad might be placed in a control group that does not get any of the drug being tested, for the term of the study.

Usually studies last eighteen months, and individuals can decline during the intervening time. It should also be noted also, however, that individuals in any study do get medical oversight. The medical personnel adhere to a protocol designed to assure the health benefits of the experiment's participants as well as noting the effectiveness, or not, of the drug being tested. These medical professionals are not the volunteer's primary care physician and problems that arise, unrelated to the study, will not be addressed by the medical group. If there is a problem or side effect of which the medical team becomes aware, they are responsible for reporting it so a decision can be made if the participant should remain in the study or if their particular problem violates the study's protocol. For instance, a gentleman who signed up for a study had an incident of malignant hypertension. When he signed up for the study, his blood pressure was normal and he had not been treated for a history of high blood pressure. Unfortunately the drug being tested was contra-indicated with high blood pressure medication. The participant had to be dropped from the study.

None of the drugs currently on the market will cure any kind of dementia. That is, they will not stop or reverse the progress of the illness. In some people, Aricept, Namenda, Exelon, Razadyne (formerly Reminyl) or Cognex may help slow the progression of the disease for a limited amount of time. Progression, though, is relentless and continues regardless of any mitigating steps taken. The best you can hope for is to slow down the progression of the disease to give you and your loved one more time together, and possibly more quality to that time. The effectiveness of any given drug also depends upon how the drug is tolerated by the individual receiving it and how susceptible they are to side effects. Remember that in taking any drug, even if it is needed, there will be side effects. While some patients' symptoms can improve dramatically, as many as half the patients taking a drug for their Alzheimer's experience no noticeable improvement.

Most of the drugs mentioned above have web sites and can be looked up online. (I have included a list in the appendix that gives individuals a place to begin to research information. I recommend printing out any useful information you find, and taking it to your loved one's physician, who can determine which drugs may be helpful in that particular case.) All medication changes should be discussed with the primary physician or his/her neurologist. Some of the information I encountered was confusing and esoteric. Again, the caution: *if what you are finding sounds too good to be true, it probably is.* It is an unfortunate fact of life that there are a lot of people out there just looking for someone whose judgment may be clouded by suffering or a desire to help.

I now come to advertisements as seen on TV that claim to help Alzheimer's. I truly want to scream every time I see one because they are so exaggerated. I imagine someone who has a mother or father with this illness seeing one of these ads and thinking, "here is an answer!" The ad may show a man or woman, unresponsive to input from their children or grandchildren—the grandchildren are the heart breakers—the voice-over (sponsor) touts their product and the next image you see is the whole family having a great time and mother or father is present with all their faculties restored, enjoying those same grandchildren. Although the verbal disclaimers are given in the voice over—no drug is for everyone—some people may be allergic or have different responses. If a picture is worth a thousand words, those pictures show the older person better, and that is what is remembered. Not only better, but back to where they were with all their faculties intact; this simply is not true. Aricept, Namenda, et al, are perfectly valid drugs, when used and prescribed at the correct time. This can be one of the difficulties; they can mitigate the rate of decline in some individuals, depending on the kind of dementia diagnosed, but these drugs never reverse dementia, only slow down the progress of the disease. One can go the web sites for these drugs and many of these sites have good information. Remember these sites are authored by and put on the internet by a drug company who wants you to minimally ask your loved one's physician about the drug. The problem comes when someone is either in denial about their loved one's condition and willing to grasp at straws, or is convinced that this drug will cure their loved one because of something they have seen on TV.

Keeping an individual with dementia on a drug for longer than is recommended can also be a problem. In our litigious society, sometimes a physician will not take someone off medication because they know the person will lose some ability. They do not want to be sued by a family for what the family may perceive as inappropriate care, even if the physician knows the person is declining and the drug is no longer effective. If one reads the research, none of the companies that make and market these drugs recommends a course of treatment with their drug in excess of three years from diagnosis. The reason they do not is because their research has shown there is no benefit after this time frame.

Another reason to take someone off an Alzheimer's drug, perhaps even early, is because every so often either the side effects warrant it or the drug causes the person to have hostility problems. While this is not common, it can and does happen.

Dementia is a terrible illness; it robs people of who they are. Families continue to hope that research will someday find a cure, but it has not yet done so.

Chapter Five

TRANSITIONS

An individual does not just come down with dementia in its most extreme form; it is a slow process and there is time to make plans and incorporate family decisions.

In the beginning you may be able to have your loved one stay at home, have caregivers come in part time, get meals on wheels and other types of short term help. If you have a large family, you may be able to share the responsibility of checking on your loved one. If the person diagnosed has a spouse, be sure that individual is on the same page as the rest of the family. Spouses have a tendency to take on more than they can do and still retain their own health, because they feel that it is their responsibility, and do not want to burden their children. Remember the spouses in question are older, too, and lack the strength that they used to have, though they will push themselves and frequently assert that they can do the job.

Another resource for the interim is adult day care. Adult day care usually runs affordable programs that give the loved one purpose and stimulation. Sometimes they have a bus service that can pick up people and drop them off at home at the end of the day. Their personnel are also an excellent resource that families can rely on, as their loved one progress further in the disease process. They will be the first to tell families when someone is no longer at a point where they fit the adult day care program. There are other resources, so be sure to be in touch with your local Alzheimer's Society.

Most communities have assisted living facilities. These can be expensive but well worth the money if it is an affordable option.

Your loved one will deteriorate. Their dementia will increase and at some point they may need a nursing home, but not out of the gate. What is recommended is staying in touch with both your loved one's primary care physician, and obtain any legal help the family may need to make whatever transitions that are coming up function smoothly, or at least as smoothly as possible.

This is like any other long term illness that one learns to live with: it can take over your life if you let it. If you do not, you can live reasonably well.

Chapter Six

KINDS OF DEMENTIA - MCI

Mild Cognitive Impairment (MCI) describes a condition that shows a person to exceed the normal levels of forgetfulness, difficulty with language, thinking and judgment for the person's age and education, yet is not at the level of a diagnosable dementia.

Individuals with MCI appear to be at risk for developing some form of dementia, but are able to stay at their current level of functioning for a very long time. In fact, they may never get worse, and the symptoms may go away. There have not been studies to determine why this happens, or how or why those individuals may improve. If your loved one has been diagnosed with MCI, all you can do is watch him or her carefully for changes and implement what- ever safety measures you feel are necessary.

This is just another reason to get your loved one to his or her physician and have tests performed. With careful monitoring your loved one may be able to stay independent and at home for a long time.

A recent study reported by the Mayo Clinic reveals that men are twice as likely to have this condition as women, and that the incidence of MCI increases with age. What is not clear is whether or not this condition leads to Alzheimer's. There appears to be no additional risk of developing some form of dementia if MCI is present. There are researchers who feel MCI may lead to Alzheimer's and others do not. Science is still out on this one. One thing is for certain, getting older is not for cowards.

Chapter Seven

KINDS OF DEMENTIA – TREATABLE ISSUES

While not really dementia, there are conditions which can mask themselves as dementia, in that they will have similar symptoms. The good news is that they are also eminently treatable. The five conditions that evidence similar symptoms are as follows: B-12 deficiency, depression, drug interactions, normal-pressure hydrocephalus and hypothyroidism.

Again, the recommendation is to go to the primary care physician immediately for diagnosis, should any of these symptoms appear. Although these are treatable issues, they must first be diagnosed, and only a physician can make that determination.

- B-12 deficiency has the following symptoms: diarrhea, numbness and tingling in hands or feet, shortness of breath, fatigue, loss of appetite, and in some cases, confusion.

Remember, all patients do not have the same symptoms or may not evidence all of them. The patient may have low B-12 levels in the blood as well as low folic acid and homocysteine levels. Once a diagnosis is made through blood chemistry, B-12 vitamins can be ordered by shot or pill and the symptoms will resolve themselves over time.

- Depression is another matter. There can certainly be a chemical imbalance, but depression can also be situational (as if a spouse dies, or simply getting older and having health problems). There appears to be a wide range of symptoms: fatigue, loss of appetite, insomnia, withdrawal from social situations, agitation, sadness, loneliness, and despair. A person may have some or all of these. An anti-depressant may be as effective for either type of depression. The kind of anti-depressant, however, is important, must be prescribed by a physician, and may require the help of cognitive therapy to fulfill its maximum potential. According to researchers, some form of cognitive therapy can help to ameliorate symptoms.

Obviously if an individual has dementia as well, medication alone is probably the way to go. A person does need a certain level of cognition in order to make talk therapy work.

• Drug interactions can have the same symptoms as depression along with occasional hallucinations. Sometimes the interaction is not between two prescribed medications, but between a prescribed medication and an over-the-counter one. It is paramount to tell your physician everything that you are putting in your body. Occasionally someone will have a side effect that is unanticipated and this can lead to problems only a physician can solve.

• Hypothyroidism is caused by the thyroid's inability to produce either enough, or in some cases, any of the thyroid hormone that our bodies need to function. The symptoms are low metabolic rate, a tendency to weight gain, mental slowness, sleepiness and sometimes myxedema (swelling that occurs around the eyes particularly, and the face in general). These symptoms are seen fairly frequently in the elderly and especially in older women. While it is not curable, a maintenance dose of thyroid hormone can be given and this is usually sufficient to take away the symptoms.

- Normal pressure hydrocephalus (NPH) is a type of hydrocephalus which can occur in older adults. NPH is different from regular hydrocephalus because it develops slowly and the parts of the brain most often affected are the memory, reasoning, problem solving, apathy, and speaking. It is often accompanied by physical signs such as a shuffling gait, falls, "freezing" while walking, and sometimes bladder control issues. NPH is caused by an increase in the cerebrospinal fluid around the brain. If this fluid cannot drain normally, it increases in pressure and causes the above symptoms.

The treatment for this condition is surgery; no other medical treatment exists. A shunt (a thin plastic tube) is implanted in the brain which allows the excess fluid to drain off. A shunt operation is not a cure and the shunt must remain in place indefinitely. It is a less than perfect solution because why this condition happens in the first place is unknown. Some individuals have the shunt installed and it does not relieve the symptoms. Along with this, there is also always the risk of infection around the shunt, and clots caused by the surgery itself. Frequently surgeons will perform a spinal tap to see if symptoms will be relieved by the decrease in spinal fluid before shunt placement.

Still, these problems can be addressed and *may* result in a reversal of the persons' symptoms. Surgery of any kind carries some risk and especially with older persons, so careful evaluation of both the treatment and results must be assessed beforehand.

Chapter Eight

KINDS OF DEMENTIA – ALZHEIMER'S

Alzheimer's dementia, or AD as it is referred to, is a progressive and fatal brain disease and the most common form of dementia known. Approximately 50-70% of all people with dementia have this kind—that amounts to about 5.3 million Americans.

Beyond memory loss, the progression of the disease slowly robs the victim of the brain processes needed for daily living. Like every part of our bodies, the brain ages and most of us are aware of slowed thinking and reaction time as this occurs. But with AD, as memory loss increases, problem-solving capabilities decrease; there is more difficulty with routine tasks and confusion with time and place.

We can only know for certain what kind of dementia a loved one my have suffered after death has occurred and an autopsy performed. We do know, that brain cells die and that plaques and tangles show up in the brains of Alzheimer patients upon autopsy. The plaques are made of beta-amyloid protein and the tangles of twisted fibers called "tau." Some how these plaques and tangles interfere with the nerve impulses traveling between neurons. We know that eventually brain cells will be killed off, beginning in the areas of memory and learning, then spreading to other regions.

New research is focused on why this happens. Scientists are trying to figure out why the plaques and tangles form and why they interfere with neuronal transmission. Unfortunately the experiments being done have, to date, conflicting results. Science is not sure if the plaques and tangles cause the disease or are simply a result of the disease process.

Behavior modification, along with input from a professional occupational therapist, appears to help AD patients at home to engage in activities of daily living better.

One note-worthy point that came from the COPE (Care of Persons with Dementia) study is that 40% of the individuals involved in the study were also diagnosed with some form of medical condition (urinary tract infections, anemia, and thyroid problems). This result supports a clear recommendation to have your loved one checked medically at least every three months, or more frequently if you see any kind of contraindication. Symptoms in the elderly can be different for the same disease process than in a younger person, or even a mature adult. For instance, some women have chronic bacteria in their urine and may require a maintenance dose of antibiotics and yet they may have no symptoms. Everything should be tested.

The Alzheimer's Association has printed on their website the Ten Warning Signs of AD, paraphrased below:

1) Marked memory loss that interrupts daily living, such as loss of notable dates and events, frequently asking for the same information, or forgetting how to do newly learned tasks.

2) Problems with planning and an inability to concentrate. They may have difficulty tracking monthly bills, or be unable to follow an often-used recipe. Persons with AD may have difficulty balancing a checkbook.

3) Difficulty with completing regular tasks, like driving to a familiar location, or

remembering the rules of an often played game.

4) Confusion with time, as in losing track of seasons, or time of day. They can also have difficulty knowing or remembering how they arrived at a place.

5) Difficulty understanding visual images, such as with reading, and judging distances (spatial relationships). The sight of their images in mirrors can be confusing.

6) Problems with written or spoken words. Inability to track and participate in a conversation. Also, word retrieval may become more difficult.

7) Losing the ability to retrace their own steps. They may hide valuable items, then accuse others of stealing those items. Persons with AD may also secret belongings in inappropriate places, like putting jewelry in the refrigerator.

8) Increase in poor judgment. People with AD may give away money or leave the stove on. Grooming may diminish.

9) A marked sign of this disease is someone withdrawing from social activities with

unreasonable excuses. This can happen early on.

10) Mood and personality changes may be evidenced. Confusion, groundless suspicion, and anxiety may be hallmarks. To feel secure in their environments, persons with AD structure specific ways of performing routines. They may become agitated if their routines get changed.

If you are seeing three or more of these symptoms, it is time to think about the problem, assist the person in seeing her primary care physician, and talk to family members about planning for the loved one's future.

Because a person does not immediately stop functioning, it is sometimes difficult to figure out what is going on. It is wise to consult other family members to see if they have noticed changes. Then, ensure the loved one goes to their physician for a chat. Be sure that the physician talks directly to the patient, not just to you. Another important thing to know is, do not argue with the person if they forget or correct you about a detail. Their reality is important, they are not making details up, they remember the occasion the way they are telling it. Make a list of symptoms you are seeing to leave with the physician and keep a log to take along that documents changes. You may need to share the log and symptom list without your loved one present. Sometimes the physician will talk directly to your loved one about necessary changes and safety, such as no longer driving, even if they still have a license.

The physician can also administer a Mini-mental Exam which tests several areas:

- Orientation: Day, date, year, month, season, place (where the person is physically at the time), floor of a building, city, county and state (1 point for each correct answer—total 10 points).
- Recall and Short term memory: Name three ordinary items (pen, ring, lamp) or any three familiar items (1 point for each correct answer—total 3 points.)
- See if the person can remember the same items three minutes later (1 point for each correct answer —total 3 points.
- Concentration: Count backwards from 100 by 7's at least five numbers—93,86,79,

72, 65. Or spell WORLD backwards. (5 points for the correct answers).

• Can the person follow a multiple command? Pick up paper with right hand, fold paper in half, put the paper on the floor or table with left hand. (1 point for each correct answer—total 3 points).

• Language: Show a sentence on paper and tell the person to do what it says:

Close your eyes (1 point correct answer).

Write a simple sentence. (1 point correct answer).

• Identify common items the tester points to: Two items. (1point correct answer—total 2 points).

• Repeat a simple sentence read to the person by tester. (1 point correct answer).

• Eye/hand coordination: Copy drawing of two intersecting five-sided figures. (1 point for correct answer). Then add up all the points.

Score of 28—30 is considered normal

Score of 26—28 has signs of mild dementia or MCI

Score of 20—26 mild dementia

Score of 10—20 moderate dementia

Score greater than 10 indicates severe dementia

Per the research, there is no guaranteed way to avoid getting AD or any other dementia. So far, it seems to be a question of good or bad luck. What we do know is that physical activity, a heart-healthy diet, and cognitive engagement helps to avoid or delay the onset of problems.

Chapter Nine

KINDS OF DEMENTIA – LEWY BODY

A diagnosis of dementia with Lewy bodies cannot be made with 100% accuracy until a post-mortem autopsy, even though it is the third most common form of dementia. However, some physicians can, through the use of an MRI, make a fairly accurate assessment. This form of dementia is often misdiagnosed, partially because it shares some characteristics of both Alzheimer's and Parkinson's. The onset of Lewy Body Dementia is typically between the ages of 60 and 80, with males at greater risk. The disease progresses rapidly and fluctuates in its progressive course, with an average life expectancy of about six years after diagnosis.

Key features of this kind of dementia include fluctuating cognitive ability, variations in attention and alertness, episodic delirium, and vivid, well-formed visual hallucinations. Extrapyramidal symptoms, such as rigidity of movement or repeated falls, along with fainting, and a transient loss of consciousness may also be present. Sensitivity to neuroleptic medications may also be an important indication of this illness, as remedies sometimes prescribed appropriately to treat hallucinations can set off a severe reaction in an individual with Lewy Body Dementia. Family members need to be aware that the drug Haloperidol (which is often given in hospital to mitigate hallucinations) can lead to a severe reaction with increased extrapyramidal symptoms in a person with Lewy Body Dementia. If your loved one is taken to the hospital, be sure to go with them and tell the attending physician that the patient may have dementia with Lewy bodies.

Being able to distinguish delirium from dementia is important. Any individual can become delirious regardless of age.

DELIRIUM SYMPTOMS:

- Sudden onset—taking hours or days to show up.
- Slurred speech
- Person goes in/out of consciousness, and can be inattentive or easily distracted
- Frequent vivid hallucinations

- Anxiety, fearfulness, suspicion or agitation
- Signs of medical illness—fever, chills, drug side effect

DEMENTIA SYMPTOMS:

- Slow onset over months or years
- Normal way of speaking
- Memory loss
- Language difficulties—both in speech and understanding
- Hallucinations—but not in every case
- Listless or apathetic mood, and/or agitation

The elderly can have delirium reactions post-surgery, and be normal again by the next day. They can frequently remember what they felt or said. It is always important to remember that no matter what the reason, when someone is having a hallucination, not to argue with them. Denying their reality is an exercise in frustration for both of you. Go along for now, correct them when they clear up.

Melinda Fengel, RN, BSN

I was just coming on duty and had been assigned a patient newly returned from surgery. She was a woman about fifty-five or so, with gray hair kept in place by a hair net. As I walked into the room to assess her condition, she said, "Thank God you're here. I can't get anyone to put the vegetables away and they will go bad." I picked up a grocery sack of magazines from her over-bed table and stuffed them in the closet. She was then happy, and I could assess her. The next afternoon she asked me if she had done anything "strange." I advised her that she had, but assured her it was a normal side effect of the pain medication she was given, and that we, as nurses, saw this all the time. I advised her not to worry about it, at which point we both had a good laugh!

Chapter Ten

FRONTOTEMPORAL, PICKS AND PROGRESSIVE APHASIA

Frontotemporal dementia describes a clinical condition in which the shrinking of the frontal and anterior temporal lobes of the brain occurs. According to the National Institute of Neurological Disorders and Stroke, this kind of dementia has a strong genetic component and FTD often runs in families. The usual lifespan is from two to ten years, after diagnosis. It is also an early onset dementia, which means the condition begins earlier than fifty years of age. Eventually, the person with this kind of dementia will need 24-hours-a-day care and monitoring.

There are two general clinical patterns to this illness; one affects behavior and the other language. Changes in behavior feature either impulsive behaviors, or bored, apathetic ones. Impulsive behavior is an indicator of inappropriate social contacts. Hallmarks are increased interest in sex, increased distractibility, agitation and sometimes changes in food preferences. Apathetic behavior features a lack of empathy, blunted emotions, and neglect of personal hygiene.

Language disturbances are characterized by difficulty in making or understanding speech. People evidencing this phase of the illness retain spatial skills and memory.

The several kinds of frontotemporal dementias are a challenge to identify precisely because the symptoms are individual and diagnosis cannot be confirmed until autopsy. They are included here because the best care comes from an accurate clinical diagnosis. Because there is a genetic component to these illnesses, genetic testing can aid families in planning.

PICK'S DISEASE

Pick's disease is a rare neurodegenerative disease that causes the progressive destruction of nerve cells in a person's brain. This disease does not have a genetic component and does not run in families. The symptoms that hallmark this illness are difficulty with speech and thinking, and changes in personality. These symptoms can show up as early as age fifty-five. The symptoms, that allow doctors to differentiate between Picks and Alzheimer's, illustrate that with Alzheimer's memory loss shows up first. With Picks disease, uncharacteristic, impulsive behaviors show up first. Diagnosis is confirmed by autopsy and the presence of Pick bodies, which is caused by the aggregation of tau (spherical) proteins in the neurons.

PRIMARY PROGRESSIVE APHASIA

Primary progressive aphasia is a rare neurological disorder that impairs both the ability to make and to understand spoken language. It can be confused with early onset Alzheimer's, but the persons affected may be able to care for themselves for as much as ten years or so after diagnosis. Some individuals become mute, other persons come to rely on sign language to communicate.

Primary progressive aphasia is caused by atrophy of the language center, in the central part of the brain's left hemisphere. Exhibited symptoms can be difficulty with word finding, difficulty naming objects, difficulty with written or spoken language, as well as misuse of words and their endings or tenses.

Taking care of someone with this kind of illness can be challenging, but with planning, a doable exercise.

Chapter Eleven

PARKINSON'S AND HUNTINGTON'S DISEASES

I have included Parkinson's in this book for a couple of reasons. It is a brain disease, and like Alzheimer's, it comes on slowly and is difficult to diagnose. Also as the disease progresses, the person who has the disease will exhibit a form of dementia.

The signs for Parkinson's are a tremor on one side, which gets worse on that same side as the disease progresses; a slowing of motion; the retardation of the ability to initiate motion; muscle rigidity; impaired balance and posture; a lack of facial expression; loss of arm swinging when walking; decreased blinking; and changes in speech, such as slurring or no speech at all.

The symptoms arise from a lack in the brain of a chemical messenger called dopamine. This neurotransmitter is responsible for sending signals that aid in coordination and balance. The lack of a chemical messenger occurs because certain cells in the brain lose their ability to produce dopamine. Science does not know why this happens, though there are many medical theories.

The risk factors for Parkinson's are age (mid-life and on), heredity, gender (more men are affected), and exposure to toxins.

No definitive test exists for Parkinson's, so it is diagnosed by a process of elimination until the later stages, when symptoms exacerbate and become obvious. There are several drugs that can be prescribed to help alleviate the symptoms, but there is no cure. Carbo/levodopa (Sinamet), currently the most successful of the Parkinsonian drugs prescribed, can be toxic to some people. Side effects may include confusion, delusions and/or hallucinations, as well as diskinesia (involuntary movements). If these side effects occur, the dosing may be changed or a different drug tried.

Although Parkinson's is a long term illness, which can be mitigated with drugs, no cure currently exists and it will eventually be fatal to the person.

Huntington's disease is addressed here because it is also a disorder of the brain and spinal cord. Huntington's is a genetic disease and people born with it have a defective gene, though symptoms often do not evidence themselves until the person is over thirty-five. Problems with balance, jerky movements, muscle weakness and mild personality changes may occur. Eventually this disease can take away a person's ability to walk, talk or swallow. A form of dementia can also occur in the later stages.

Genetic testing is recommended if you have someone in your family with Huntington's. Genetic counseling is available to provide advice and guidance throughout the process. Though currently there is no cure for Huntington's, early testing provides individuals with time to plan and make arrangements if one is positive for this defective gene. Stem-cell research has provided some positive results, but science is still working on a cure.

Chapter Twelve

KINDS OF DEMENTIA – KORSAKOFF'S SYNDROME

Alcohol is a drug. It may be a legal drug and a socially acceptable drug, but it is a drug nonetheless. Taken in sufficient quantities over time, it can cause Korsakoff's Syndrome or Alcohol Related Dementia.

Basically it is a neurological disorder caused by a lack of thiamine (vitamin B1) in the brain. The two conditions precipitating this vitamin deficiency are chronic alcoholism and severe malnutrition. Science can help some of the symptoms via replacement therapy, but the damage done to the thalamus and the mammillary bodies of the hypothalamus, as well as generalized cerebral atrophy, is irreversible. It should be noted that vitamin B1 replacement therapy only works on someone who is no longer drinking any alcohol of any kind.

The symptoms of Korsakoff's are the following:

Confabulation – invented memories which are believed by the person due to gaps in real memory; sometimes this tendency is due to blackouts

Long and short term memory loss

Meager conversational content

Lack of insight

Apathy

The first issue to be considered is whether the person can or will stop drinking. Are they willing to be detoxed? Frequently, individuals who have been drinking for years require medical detoxification. Even if people have been only maintenance drinkers, their bodies are saturated with alcohol. Is the person in question a candidate for a rehabilitation program? Has his or her dementia sufficiently progressed that stopping drinking is pointless? Will the person return to drinking given the opportunity? Are all family members aware and on the same page? Because if not, the drinker may get one friend or family member to smuggle booze to him, no matter where he is.

Sometimes a family has given up on a loved one because they have been unable to affect a change in the person's alcohol behavior. Then the loved one gets dementia, and the family must try to cope with the person who has both an alcohol problem and dementia.

As a family you must decide the best course of action.

In the community where I worked, only one person was brought in who had been chemically detoxed. This family had elected to make their loved one clean and sober. The gentleman in question was very bright and continually thought up reasons I should give him a drink. Every day he had a new idea, but his favorite repetitive saying was, "You're a nurse. Why do you need some doctor telling you what to do?"

I always responded the same way, "My job depends on my keeping the rules and if your doctor orders me to give you a drink and your family will bring in your drink of choice, I will see that you get it."

Day after day he would come to me with endless excuses about why he should have a drink, and regardless of what his doctor said, I should do what he wanted. His dementia not withstanding, he remembered he wanted a drink, even if he couldn't remember eating lunch.

More than once his family, or one of our caregivers, found vodka and other alcohol in his refrigerator. They always took the alcohol away, but it took some investigation on everyone's part to discover that it was a grandson who was bringing him in his supply. In an effort to please him his family brought in non-alcoholic beer to keep in his refrigerator, and this appeared to satisfy him. Still, on occasion, he would ask me to get him a cocktail.

Alcohol confounds and exacerbates dementia. Families who have a loved one with both issues are looking at an overwhelming task, and need professional help in order to solve the problems.

Chapter Thirteen

VASCULAR DEMENTIA

Vascular dementia occurs when blood flow to the brain stops for either a long or short time. When it happens short term it is called a transient ischemic attack (TIA). The effects frequently disappear with in minutes or hours, and leave the person with no perceptible difficulties. Dementia occurs when these mini-strokes happen over time and go unnoticed, but because more and more of the brain areas become damaged, the symptoms of vascular dementia begin to appear. There are several different types of brain system failings.

- Small vessel disease, or a mixture of TIAs and small vessel disease, can cause vascular dementia. It is the second most common type of dementia after Alzheimer's.

- There are actually two kinds of strokes. Ischemic strokes occur when a blood vessel supplying the brain becomes blocked. It can be blocked by a blood clot, or cholesterol (fat) that collects in the arteries, forming plaque. A piece breaks off and clogs an artery. The second kind of stroke is hemorrhagic where a vessel becomes weak and bursts open causing a bleed into the brain area. This kind of stroke is generally caused by an aneurysm or arteriovenous malformation.

- A cerebral vascular accident (CVA) is a medical emergency and should be treated immediately. TIA's should be seen to by a physician, even if the symptoms have disappeared. The risk factors for having a CVA are high blood pressure, atrial fibrillation, diabetes, family history of stroke, high cholesterol, increasing age over fifty-five, race (black people are more likely to have a CVA) and heart disease.

There are life styles which put people at risk, such as being overweight, drinking heavily, eating a lot of fat and salt, smoking, or taking illegal drugs.

The reverse is also true. If you minimize your life style choices, you can cut your risk factors, particularly as you age. That does not mean you can do what you want as a young person, then behave once you are older. The same factors that are recommended for a heart-healthy life style, apply here; exercise, lose weight, keep your brain active. Take high blood pressure or cholesterol medication as your physician prescribes. If you must drink, do it with moderation. Give up smoking. Reduce the amount of fat and salt eaten. Do not do illegal drugs.

There is no magic to avoid stroke or vascular dementia, and doing all the right things is no guarantee that you will not have a CVA. But you can reduce the risk.

If you have a loved one diagnosed with vascular dementia, get that person to his or her physician and follow the prescribed regimen. If science cures heart disease, rates of vascular dementia will drop markedly.

Chapter Fourteen

STAGES OF DEMENTIA

Staging systems are useful frameworks for understanding how the disease process may unfold. I say "may unfold," because each individual is different and his or her disease process will be individual as well. It should be noted that "staging" refers only to Alzheimer's, and does not take into account other forms of dementia, such as Lewy Body or Pick's Disease.

Many experts have documented common patterns that occur in individuals with Alzheimer's. Staging is a way of generalizing the process of the disease, which follows the progression of symptoms. Remember that any individual may have a symptom or two from more than one category at a given time, and when a person is staged, it is a compilation of factors that places a person in a particular category.

- Stage I: No cognitive impairment. Individuals are unimpaired, showing no memory problems or functional problems. No problems are evident to a medical professional.

- Stage II. Very mild cognitive decline. Individuals are aware of memory problems, words and names get lost, losing familiar objects—like glasses—occurs, and perhaps loss in some areas of function. These issues may not be evident to medical assessment, but are frequently noticed by family, friends and co-workers.

- Stage III. Mild cognitive decline. Re-asking the same questions only a short while after being given an answer. Friends and family become concerned with problems of concentration, word-finding, decreased ability to interact with friends and family, and performance issues in social settings. When reading a passage or article, the individual may retain little meaning, or the person may misplace valuable objects. Also noticeable may be a decline in the person's ability to plan and organize. Problems are very evident on medical examination.

- Stage IV: Moderate cognitive decline. At this stage, medical interviews detect clear-cut deficits. Signs of this stage are decreased knowledge of current events, impaired ability to perform mentally challenging drills (as in arithmetic or backwards spelling), decreased capacity to perform shopping or dinner planning, difficulties dealing with finances, or exhibiting reduced time-inaccurate memory of personal history. In some individuals incontinence can begin, or exacerbate.

- Stage V: Moderately severe cognitive decline. At this stage there are major gaps in memory and deficits in cognitive function. Some assistance with activities of daily living can become essential. Symptoms of confusion become apparent, such as where they are, what they should do, or what is next in their routine. Individuals can have trouble with choosing clothing for the season (they may put on summer clothes in the winter), they may require assistance with toileting or changing their briefs. They may change clothing many times during the day for no apparent reason, or pack up their room to leave. They may feel they are in a different time in their lives and ask for a long dead husband or children of school age. They may have hallucinations, think dreams are real, and exhibit personality changes.

- Stage VI: Severe cognitive decline: Memory difficulties increase and sometimes individuals lose their surroundings (not know where they are, or think they are another place), forget the names of familiar people, need help with all activities of daily living, incidents of increased incontinence, fecal incontinence, disruption of sleep cycle, and forgetting of family members like grandchildren. They tend to wander without purpose. Hearing aids and dentures become annoying. If not removed from view, these items are liable to get thrown away in a tissue.

- Stage VII: Very severe cognitive decline: Individuals may lose the ability to speak or hold conversations. Frequently they lose the ability to walk without assistance, may need to be fed, may have difficulty swallowing, may not be able to hold up their heads. If in bed, to avoid skin breakdown, they must be turned and repositioned every two hours.

One must remember that there are other factors that affect a person's ability to perform actions, such as walking. These other disease processes affecting their physical abilities will be concomitant to their dementia.

Staging is useful when speaking to medical professionals or intake personnel of a care facility where one is considering placing a loved one. There are no absolutes, but this should be considered a valuable tool.

Chapter Fifteen

A PSYCHIATRIST'S STORY

Early in my nursing career, I worked in a hospital on the orthopedic and neurology floor. This meant that we took care of all the broken hips, or hip replacements, knee replacements, strokes and people with seizures. It also meant that many of the individuals who made up our population were older folks, and sometimes the person we were assigned to take care of had dementia. Since we cared for a lot of older patients, I thought it incumbent upon me to learn what I could about dementia. What follows is a story I was told in a seminar, which was authored by an advocacy group, to increase nurses' understanding of dementia and the concomitant problems faced by those who provided care to patients.

The mother of a female psychiatrist, Dr. Baum, resided in a nursing home, the only alternative available at the time. Dr. Baum visited every night after work, knowing that her mother would receive exceptional care if she checked on her regularly. In those days, there were no units strictly catering to the care of a person with dementia. Besides having dementia, her mother was wheelchair bound and required a lot of physical care.

Running late one night, the doctor hurried to the nurses station when her mother wasn't in her room as expected. At the desk, the on-duty nurse said that her mother was in the solarium. Dr. Baum hurried down the hall, her normal guilt compounded by being late. She was sure her mother would not only miss her and be aware she was late, but would probably be put off by "coming in second," to Dr. Baum's work--a complaint her mother had leveled at her in the past. As the doctor reached the solarium, she paused and silently opened the double door—all the while trying to think of a viable excuse—the traffic, a place to park, etc.—when she became aware of two people talking. The wheelchairs of two elderly patients were about three feet apart, facing one another, with a small table near her mother's hand. But what struck the doctor was what was happening between the two women in the wheelchairs. First, one would speak then she would politely wait for the other woman to reply. They laughed together at what appeared to be the appropriate places in the conversation. There was only one catch. Dr. Baum's mother, having lost her secondary language, was speaking Yiddish and the other lady was speaking Japanese.

The lessons the psychiatrist took from this encounter were three-fold. First, people can communicate even without language, and communication is the glue that holds us together. Second, peer interaction can distract and fulfill a resident with dementia. Third, guilt is a wasted emotion. Her mother no longer had a reference for time passed. Her mother was not aware her daughter was late, she was just glad to see her. To be accurate, her mother had used guilt as a tool before her illness, but was no longer capable of doing so.

The doctor's admonition to the nurses listening to her story was "be sure to tell families that they do not have to respond to the old tapes of their parents voices in their heads." A person with dementia is not the person they remember from their childhood; this person has neither the positive nor negative attributes they exhibited in their earlier years. Take them as they come. If they are negative, deflect; if they are positive, enjoy! As long as your loved one is alive and capable of joyful moments, indulge them and yourself.

Chapter Sixteen

DRUGS

Drugs can be miraculous, but they need to be carefully tracked, not just to see if they do the job for which they were intended, but also to determine if the side effects are tolerable or make the person taking them even sicker. One needs to remember that side effects are not what *will* happen, but what *could* happen when one takes a particular drug. While looking up a drug on the internet is commendable, it is important to understand what you are reading, and be aware that the drug company that made the drug is giving you the information.

Another thing to remember is that any given person's system may not conflict with a specific drug, and so not respond appropriately. For instance, some people can take penicillin for a bacterial infection, others must take erythromycin, a different antibiotic, because penicillin is ineffective for them or they may have an allergic reaction to it. The reverse is true as well. Any person could find erythromycin ineffective or not be able to deal with the side effects, while tolerating penicillin just fine.

Someone with dementia should be watched closely both for the intended drug effect and for side effects. They cannot tell you when they have a problem. They can act out, however. Physicians cannot know what will happen and must rely on family and caregivers to report back to them about what they are seeing, particularly when a new drug is added to a dementia resident's regimen.

One question to ask is, what kind of drug is being given and what should one see? If the drug is a blood pressure medication, the person's blood pressure should be taken weekly to assess the effect (to determine if the blood pressure went down). If the physician is unsure of what is causing a particular problem, your loved one's blood pressure may need to be taken daily or even several times per day. This way the titration (dose by weight) of the drug will be more accurate.

Also it is important to keep in mind that some drugs take longer to work than others. Drugs, like antibiotics, work fairly quickly within forty-eight to seventy-two hours. The effects of antidepressants may be four to six weeks out. Be sure you ask the physician what to expect and when to expect it. If you do not see the result you think you should, provide feedback to the physician so he or she can try a different drug or a different dose.

Even when someone has been on a medication for a long time, her body may change, so monthly vitals for a dementia resident—even who appears to be stable--are important. Things can change. Vital signs are called "vital signs" for a reason. This is the first place a change will occur when something is amiss. Vital signs should be taken weekly if your loved one is given a new drug, and all symptom changes should be reported to the physician immediately.

That said, one needs to think of any product someone uses as a medication. When dementia begins, a person with symptoms may use over- the-counter medications or vitamins appropriately, but as the dementia progresses they will not. Remember products that have different goals have different ingredients. For instance, many body lotions contain alcohol and are marked for external use only. One dementia resident put lotion on her teeth thinking they would get white because the lotion was white. Another lady put something (we are not sure what) all over her face. The skin on her face turned red and became swollen. We could never determine what she used because she could not tell us. We called her primary physician and he gave us an order for oral Benadryl which helped. Her family took all the lotions, potions, and cleaning products out of her room. They locked away all her things and let her use some items, only with either a family member or caregiver present. It needs to be noted that Benadryl is frequently used for allergies, but certain individuals can be allergic to this as well, or they might be taking another drug that is contraindicated with Benadryl, so its use should be cleared with the physician.

All over-the-counter medications, lotions, shampoo, toothpaste, makeup and many other items need to be looked at for safety considerations. Individuals progress in their dementia and while keeping them as independent as possible is important, keeping them safe is critical.

It is foreseeable that when someone's dementia changes, the person may use an item (previously used appropriately) in an incorrect manner. Therefore, it behooves families to buy products that are as benign as possible. Completely natural products, that may be ideal, can be found through the internet, or at the local health food store. Still, my recommendation is to keep available items to a minimum and allow the use of some products with either family or caregiver supervision.

There was a lady—who was probably a Stage 3 —who insisted she could keep Extra Strength Tylenol by her bedside in case she woke up in the night in pain. She could have called for the same pill, but both her family and her physician felt she could do this safely. One night she woke up, did not turn on the light, reached over for the pill she knew was there, and her glass of water, and swallowed her hearing aide. The next morning when she realized what she had done, she called her family. They had quite the job looking for her hearing aide, which found, cleaned and fixed so she could wear it again.

In addition, when any drug is given to an elderly person, it is important to understand that there may be age-related changes that alter the therapeutic or toxic effect of that drug.

As we age, the proportion of fat to lean mass and water quantity changes. Lean mass decreases while fat mass increases--even in people who are not overweight--and in women that change tends to be even greater. Body makeup varies from one person to the next, but the body changes that do happen can alter the relationship between a drug's concentration and its distribution in the body.

For instance, a water-soluble drug may stay in the blood stream longer because there is less lean body mass. Elderly patients may also have greater difficulty absorbing drugs than younger patients. This can be a significant problem if the drug has a narrow therapeutic range.

Drugs are wonderful things, but should be used with forethought and caution.

Chapter Seventeen

BEHAVIORS

As dementia progresses, and even when the first symptoms are noticed, behavior can be a problem that may or may not require medication.

Behavior is frequently telling us something. Of course there is a problem, but frequently that problem is fear. The person with the oncoming dementia knows something is different and is unsure of what to do about it. This fear can then produce agitation and acting out. The two most helpful tools to use are *distraction* and *redirection*. Distraction can take a lot of forms, but basically requires getting the person with dementia involved in something to aid in forgetting the agitation. A cup of tea, a walk, just talking about the leaves on the trees or the flowers can be distracting. Saying, "let us go do x," whatever x is, directs attention to something else. Suggesting task, like folding clean linen, may help the person to feel useful, and can precipitate a decrease of anxiety.

When dealing with parents, try doing whatever it was they did for you, to help you cope, when you were a child and upset with life. Suggest a hot cup of cocoa or a warm bath. Give them a gentle stroke on the shoulder, a kind word, or just take the time to listen to what is frightening them. People with dementia are scared because they no longer have the tools to ameliorate a problem, they cannot "think it through."

If the person is having hallucinations, find out if it is scary or benign, because what you want to do in response is different. If it is benign, ask for a description of it. If the loved one just wants you to fix it, tell him or her you will and suggest in the meantime you both have a cup of tea, or a glass of milk.

There was a lady who kept seeing people she didn't know in her apartment. Because she could still use the phone, she would call my office and ask me to come up and have the people removed. I would go to her apartment, prop open the door, and suggest aloud that the people leave. If they didn't disappear, I would suggest that she take a walk with me while her guests left, giving her time to forget. All this does take time, lots of time, so if you use caregivers, be certain that they understand that you want them to pay attention to your loved one. Paying attention is a caregiver's most important task, and anything else they do is secondary. Tasks can always get done; people cannot wait.

People with dementia can sometimes tell you when they have pain, but not always. Frequently, pain is at the basis of acting out. As people age bones and muscles can hurt from any number of problems. Sometimes a couple of Tylenol will help, and sometimes they need a prescription drug. Remember, to a person with dementia, pain is total. Like children, they cannot reason, they just hurt. While the physician is the appropriate person to prescribe medication, the person with dementia may tell the physician they have no pain. At the moment, that is what is true and they don't remember twenty minutes ago. You must be the advocate, keeping track of when they complain of pain, how often and to what degree. For instance, are you seeing them grimace when they sit or stand? Do they cry out when moving a particular limb? Is there something you or they can do to relieve the discomfort besides taking medication? The use of ice or heat can be beneficial. The only reason an individual should be medicated for pain is if the pain is causing suffering. You need to keep on hand whatever it takes to relieve pain when it occurs.

If every distraction fails and the person is still miserable with anxiety, a visit to their physician is a must to obtain the appropriate medication. Once a medication is tried, it is up to you to see what the consequences are, and if there are side effects. You must be the eyes and ears of the physician and report back to him so he knows if what he is suggesting, is working. Often a good way to do this is via e-mail, if the physician has one. Otherwise a weekly report should be sent to the physician so it can become a part of your loved one's records. You are his or her best advocate!

Another time medication is necessary is if the person becomes violent. When a person is violent with or without dementia, they are operating on adrenaline and not capable of controlling their actions. To prevent injury to themselves and others, they must be medicated. If anger and violent behavior become a pattern, the person may require a stay in a geriatric unit that specializes in psychiatric help for the elderly. Unfortunately, this need is not all that unusual when you are dealing with a person with dementia. Sometimes a medication will minimize behaviors until the disease progresses to a further stage, and it is no longer needed.

Remember that when behavior indicates some form of distress, it is up to you and the doctor to be detectives and figure it out.

Chapter Eighteen

LEGAL ISSUES

States vary widely in their requirements and restrictions regarding what documents to submit and which procedures must be followed—if a family needs to take control of assets—once your mother or father is diagnosed with dementia. Even before a formal diagnosis is made, it is a good idea to sit down with your parents and discuss their wishes, in case they lack the capacities to express their desires, at some point in time.

Few people look forward to having this discussion. Often the parent does not want to have it because signifies the potentiality of losing of control. You can assure them that none of this goes into effect unless they become incapacitated.

Money, and the potential power it brings, can do some very strange things to individuals and families. I have heard enough stories to know that this often comes as a surprise to someone trying to do the right thing. Family dynamics can sometimes fracture families, particularly if one party does not see a problem in the same way others experience the situation.

In an effort to involve and appease some family members, I have seen people wait too long, until the court must become involved in order to straighten it all out. Sometimes a court is the answer, but mediation may be tried first.

A woman named Bess, who had dementia, lived at our facility. Bess had two daughters, Claire and Deena. While Claire came to see her mother regularly, Deena did not. Claire never asked her mother about her finances or anything else, as she did not want to impose on her. Deena's son, Floyd, came to see Bess on occasion, but not often. During one of his visits, Floyd told Bess he could live in her house as long as she felt she would live in the facility. That way a family member would be there to look after her things. He then asked Bess to sign papers to that effect. She did. Bess did not understand she was signing over her house and more than fifty acres. According to Claire, Bess had planned to sell the acreage to finance her stay in a facility once she ran out of ready cash. Bess was close to 100 years old and eventually she did run out of money. When the bookkeeper advised Claire that her mother's money was gone, Claire attempted to sell her mother's house and property. Claire discovered the house and property were already gone. Deena as the eldest daughter then took charge and put her mother in a nursing home because that was what could be covered by Bess' Medicare income. There was nothing Claire could do about it.

If at all possible, it is a good idea to sit down with your loved ones before anything happens. Get them to designate a child, or children, who can speak for them in case that they cannot speak for themselves. This is not a bad idea for anyone, regardless of age and mental status. Make a list of things which are acceptable and not acceptable to them, if they become incapacitated. To what extent do they wish the family to go, if an illness appears to be mutable? To someone in their thirties, there does not seem anything worse than death, but by the time she is in her fifties, there may be a whole list of things that are worse than dying. Everyone's ideas about what those items might be are different.

Some states require an easy to ready form called a POLST—Physicians Order for Life-Sustaining Treatment. A POLST is a short form of a living will which spells out what should be done if a person requires the attention of EMT's. Currently there are eleven states where this is required, and fifteen more states that are working on enacting a POLST. The argument for having this document on file is that when emergency personnel are called in, it is easy to figure out what should be done for the patient. The down side is that the information in the document is very general and does not focus upon some issues, which can only be addressed by an attorney, in a living will. What tends to happen is that the POLST replaces the living will. It is best to have both. If someone has a living will, it should be on file with the person's primary care physician's office and the local hospital. This ensures that if the EMT's are called, the person's wishes will be taken into consideration. Each person should have a designated Health Care Proxy as well, a person who knows someone's choices and can make Health Care decisions.

The first section of the POLST asks if a person wishes to be resuscitated if the heart stops beating. Frequently the first and automatic answer is yes, but with patients who have dementia, the question to ask is what are they being saved for? Are they going to get better or worse if they come out of this trauma? A person with dementia always declines after a trauma of any kind. In addition, there is the issue of cardio/pulmonary resuscitation itself. Ribs are almost always broken in the act of compressions. CPR efficacy is questionable unless used with an electro/cardio stimulator. CPR alone, except in cases of near drowning, almost always fails.

The POLST should be filled out by a family in concert with their M.D., so that the different sections can be explained properly, and choices made from a place of knowledge, rather than guessing.

If it is affordable, get an appointment with an Elder Attorney and pick her brain about the options. Even if you cannot afford to have an attorney do all the work, a single meeting with one can give you great direction and let you know what to pursue, and what not to bother with. Be sure to make a list of questions and concerns for him so that no one's time is wasted. Remember, he does not know your family and you are asking for advice while only giving him a thumbnail sketch of the issues. Elder Law is the legal practice of counseling and representing older people and their representatives about the legal aspects of health and long-term care planning, public benefits, surrogate decision-making, and an older person's legal capacity. They also assist with the disposition and administration of estates. The purpose of certification is to identify lawyers who have enhanced knowledge, skills, and experience to be properly identified as Elder Law attorneys.

Do not put off talking to your parent(s) and/or siblings. This may be a one-person job, but it should not be a one-person decision. Siblings have strong feelings, and hashing out what is proper care for a loved one is not a one meeting drill. If everyone is not on the same page, you can get both legal and counseling help, but these issues need to be clarified and planned for, before they occur. Mediation is always another alternative and mediators can be found through the courts.

As people live longer and physically healthier lives, it becomes clear that all of us need to plan, to avoid hassles and difficulties in the future.

Chapter Nineteen

LIVING YOUR OWN LIFE: JUNE'S STORY

While this lady's story is unique, I have learned that everyone is different and all the stories have lessons from which we can all benefit.

This particular lady, I will call "June," lost her husband, Gordon, when he was sixty-three and she was sixty-one. Having been married for forty years, and having raised three children to productive citizenship, June felt it was important to focus her energy on those matters near and dear to her heart. In other words, to build a new life for herself, separate and apart from the interests of her children.

Prior to his death, Gordon had had a weak heart from having rheumatic fever as a child, and had been seeing his physician about his condition. They had discussed multiple bypass surgery, but the procedure, at the time, was not all that common and before he could implement a plan to fix his heart, he died of a massive heart attack. June believed that the way her husband died was a blessing under the circumstances. She was a consummate realist and knew Gordon would rather die than live crippled, with less than his usual quality of life.

After her husband was gone, June cut her hair into a fashionable bob, bought some new clothes, and decided she would give her time to her church, which she believed in implicitly. As a long-time, dedicated feminist, and a member of a Unitarian congregation near her home, June felt strongly that the by-laws of her church should be re-assessed. She had investigated the issue of gender bias in the church bylaws, and had decided that there should be a resolution introduced at the annual General Assembly to address the problem. Toward that end, she drafted a resolution called "Women and Religion." While a certain amount of work was done by a research committee, it was June who authored the statement, and by 1977 her petition to place the resolution on the yearly agenda was approved—it passed the General Assembly unanimously. June had virtually rewritten the seven principles by which the Unitarian Association functions. The new principles set forth: 1) the inherent worth and dignity of every person; 2) justice, equality and compassion in human relations; 3) acceptance of one another and encouragement to spiritual growth in our congregation; 4) a free and responsible search for truth and meaning; 5) the right of conscience and the use of the democratic process within the congregations and in society at large; 6) the goal of world community with peace, liberty and justice for all; and 7) respect for the interdependent web of all existence of which we are a part.

When June made the decision to move to the Pacific Northwest, it was to be near her family. After researching where she wanted to live, she picked out and moved into an assisted living community. She was adamant that she did not ever want to go into a nursing home, which she termed "a ghetto for the elderly." At that time, June also asked her daughter to take her to an attorney to organize her finances, establish a power of attorney, and dictate what she wanted done with both her money and her care, should she become incapacitated. After she had been in her apartment for over a year, June noticed that she could not come up the words she wanted. Though her daughter often knew what it was she meant, June was having trouble recalling the words she wanted to use. June was bright, she had been articulate and a writer, so not being able to come up with a particular word was both scary and frustrating.

She had taken the step of selling her car while living in the East, a full two years before moving to the Northwest. Because she didn't know the roads or where places were located, June relied on her daughter to take her on errands. .

June thoroughly loved being out of doors, because of the sensory stimulus, and since she was losing her hearing. Though she wore bi-lateral hearing aids, eventually they became more annoying than useful, and she stopped wearing them altogether. Being out of doors soothed her and simply watching nature became her passion. She would go for a walk just to enjoy the scenery. However, because she couldn't hear and couldn't say where she was going or when she intended to return due to her increasing dementia, the assisted living community wanted her to move to a more secure facility. They were concerned that she would get hurt while out alone. June's daughter ended up finding her a more secure facility and one that catered to Alzheimer's patients.

Because June realized she was "missing" pieces, she asked her physician for medication in additional to her antidepressants which she had been on for many years. June was convinced that her antidepressants were effective. Because she was so certain of this, she asked that the antidepressants be incorporated into her Health Care Request (a short enumeration of requested actions in case of emergency), and that these medications always be continued.

As time went on, June began to have falls, but did well when given a walker, even though she was in a more advanced stage of dementia. While it is always a challenge to assess where anyone is on the dementia scale, it was particularly difficult to assess what stage June was at for several reasons, not the least of which was her hearing problem and the difficulty she had finding the words she meant to say. Effectively, June's taking to walker use may have indicated she was still in an earlier stage of moderate dementia than her family thought.

Her family had never taken her to a neuropsychologist for a definitive diagnosis, and when they did take her, the diagnosis was Alzheimer's. However, the physician did not stage June.

One day June had an episode, while sitting at the dining room table. She went "blank" for about ten minutes, and then appeared to spontaneously wake up. In the meantime, 911 had been called, she was taken to ER, and her family notified. As her awakening occurred on the gurney, the Emergency Medical Techs decided that she still needed to be examined in ER. Then with no definitive determination made, she was returned to her home community. Her family realized that if she had fallen and, perhaps broken a hip, she would have to be transported to ER, but if she was not hurt, or in need of medical help, they did not want her to be transported. She was incapable of answering questions and would only be further confused by an ER experience. The community had no doctor available who would be able to make a clear determination about whether or not to transport her. The community advised her family that without proper medical intervention available, they were required by law, to call 911 if there was any kind of incident regardless of whether or not there was an obvious injury. It was the job of the EMTs to determine if she should be transported to ER and the job of the ER doctors to further assess her to determine if June should be admitted.

The only thing the family could do was publish a hand-out statement, with June's physician's blessing, asking the Emergency Medical Techs to read it before they made a decision to transport her. The statement says:

> THIS LADY HAS ASKED THAT ANTIBIOTICS AND IV'S NOT BE ADMINISTERED TO HER AND THAT SHE BE ALLOWED TO STAY IN FAMILIAR SURROUNDINGS. IF AT ALL POSSIBLE, WE ASK THAT YOU HONOR HER, AND HER PHYSICIAN'S REQUESTS FOR COMFORT MEASURES ONLY, NO ANTIBIOTICS AND NO TRANSPORTATION TO THE ER OR HOSPITAL AS INDICATED IN THE ATTACHED DOCUMENT. PLEASE PROVIDE ASSISTANCE IN HELPING THIS LADY TO HER BED. THANK YOU FOR RESPECTING THESE WISHES.

The statement was signed by her power of attorney, which in this case was her daughter. This request has been honored to date.

June's daughter takes her out for a ride once a week if the weather permits. They go somewhere for a treat—frequently a milkshake—and they enjoy their time together. It is difficult to know exactly what goes on in June's mind—what she wants or likes is truly an open question. Recently, however, when all three of her children were together on a visit to her—out of the clear blue June said, "What a treat, all three of my progeny together at the same time!" She obviously enjoyed that!

Most people with Alzheimer's go through their day getting stimulation where they can (like watching nature through the window), and interacting with those they love in whatever way they can, but every so often they will have a moment of clarity and joy!

The fact that June and her family made decisions predicated on her wishes so that she could live the life she wanted to the end of her days, is paramount. None of us knows how or when our lives will end, but it is certainly incumbent upon us to make those decisions while we can, and not leave them to others—even our family members—if at all possible. It is next to impossible for family members to get things exactly as wished; after all they are people with their own thoughts, feelings and priorities.

Chapter Twenty

DRESSING

For most people, dressing is a reflection of their personality, and that style sense goes on into old age and also into dementia—at least in the beginning. There will come a time when individuals do not know what they are putting on, do not care, and would be happy in pajamas or sweats because those clothing items are the most comfortable.

There was a lady in our facility I will call Ruth. She had been the social secretary to an influential and financially successful business executive. Even with early dementia, she dressed up everyday as if she were going to work, complete with makeup and wig. She had disliked the color of her hair when it began turning gray, and decided to wear a wig of steel gray, a color she felt set off her skin to better advantage. While her daughter and I giggled about this small vanity, we both actually admired Ruth for her sense of style. Even though her dementia increased, and though she needed more help, she was adamant about dressing up, long after most of her friends had lost their desire to wear anything but comfortable clothes.

One evening, Ruth came down for dinner in an outfit she had created. She was wearing a beige silk shirt, pajama bottoms made of a silky material in an animal pattern in tones of beige and brown. Around her neck and over her shoulders was the beige mat that went around the toilet bowl. She had draped this item carefully and crossed the arms of the mat over her chest, securing it with a topaz colored broach. She looked absolutely stunning, and proceeded into dinner, sitting and eating with great aplomb as if dressed for an event.

Usually it is easier for people with dementia to put on clothes that pull on, rather than having to deal with buttons or zippers. But the act of dressing itself may require some help. Often individuals can dress themselves if given an indication about what is wanted, and sometimes they even have preferences, but choice questions like "which outfit do you feel like wearing, the pink or the blue?" is easier for them to answer than open ended questions like, "which outfit would you like to wear?" This kind of question may not compute and may only confuse them.

There will come a time when a person with dementia will look at a piece of underwear and have absolutely no idea what to do with it. At this juncture, the person will need help with each step of dressing.

Frequently people with dementia will change their clothes for no apparent reason, perhaps several times a day. It is the caregiver's job to see that the person with dementia is, at least, dressed properly for the weather. Changing clothes may be a hassle for the person doing the caregiving, but the drill can please the person with dementia.

No one knows why individuals with dementia feel compelled to change their clothing repeatedly. It is one of the mysteries of the illness. If you ask a person with dementia why they are doing what they are doing, they can tell you they need to change, or make up some excuse to fit the situation, but they cannot answer the question.

As dementia progresses, individuals can put the wrong item on the wrong part of their body. We had a gentleman who put his legs through the arms of his sweater. When this happens, full dressing help is necessary.

We advise families who are moving a loved one into a community, to bring along fewer, rather than more, clothes. It is better to arrange the clothing in outfits so it is easier for the person with dementia to choose what to wear. Especially important is to bring along a couple of different weight sweaters and jackets, as older people feel the cold more severely. Keep the choices simple.

Chapter Twenty-one

EATING

We do not often think about the act of eating because we just do it. We eat when we feel hunger. In the western world, we often think of eating as a social function, but it is critically important to our well being. We not only need enough to eat, but also a beneficial kind of nutrition.

With dementia, eating—unless there is a mechanical problem—is something most people can do without thinking. Whether in a community or at home, a person who has dementia can sit down at a table and eat a meal. They do it correctly because they have done it all their lives. However, it is difficult for them to tell someone what they want to eat. Families will often pick up on this, if they try to take a parent with dementia out to eat. Mom or Dad will say things like, "I don't care what I eat," or "You choose for me."

What is really going on is that there are too many choices and multiple choices are confusing.

Even in a community, the people taking orders know what each resident likes and will ask them leading questions, so that the person feels like they are participating in the ordering process. The choices are actually limited.

Whether in a community or at home, individuals with dementia will be able to feed themselves, for the most part, into Stage 6 and sometimes beyond. Often, in the later stages, a well-run community will have caregivers eat with the residents, modeling appropriate behavior, and have the residents just follow along.

When a person has difficulty swallowing, that is a different story. If someone is having this problem, or you think that they might be headed this way, speak to your loved one's physician who can order a speech evaluation by a licensed speech-language therapist (SLP). The SLP can test how the person is swallowing, what difficulty they may be having. Often it can be caused by thin liquids, like drinking water when taking pills. Other times it can be a problem with the person's throat or swallowing mechanism. Whatever the case, the therapist can usually recommend changes to the person's diet (like a mechanical soft diet or finger foods) or changing their drink to thicken liquids, to help.

The danger of ignoring a swallowing difficulty is that the patient can aspirate either food or liquid into his or her lungs. That food or liquid can graduate into pneumonia. Sometimes this can happen anyway, but it is less likely once changes are made by a speech therapist.

Nutrition is another area which needs to be reviewed. All elderly do not eat as frequently or as much food as younger folks, partially because they are not doing the same level of physical activity and also because their bodies do not need the same amount of food. Their metabolism has slowed down. They do need proper nutrition, however, and their physician should recommend a good quality multiple vitamin, perhaps with minerals, depending on blood level outcomes.

The elderly have a slowed digestive mechanism. Sometimes they do not want to eat either breakfast or dinner (depending on the person). Not only is that normal, it is probably healthier for them than three meals per day. It is important that the largest meal be served midday, so that their systems have a chance to fully digest it. This is automatically done in most communities that cater to seniors because it lowers the rate of indigestion.

When their loved one is living in a community, families should provide a list to the caregivers of food likes/dislikes and food allergies or sensitivities. Also, they need to inform about the kinds of foods the person is used to eating and when he/she eats them —snacks included. One lady under our care drank a cup of hot water before every meal, and had done so for many years. She believed it kept her regular. Most communities will try to accommodate the items an individual enjoys. It makes the whole meal experience more pleasant and usual for them. Routine similarities are important.

Do not go to a big discount store and buy snacks for your loved one and put those snacks in their apartment. Be aware that a person with dementia, even early dementia, cannot remember what or when they last ate. If you bring them big bags of treats, they will eat them, often at one sitting, and sometimes not eat their meal. Treats should be given out either when the person asks, or on a timed schedule, and not left where they can be casually found by a person with dementia.

Chapter Twenty-two

TIME TRAVELERS: TOM'S STORY

A tall, gaunt gentleman named Tom was brought to
our facility by his wife, Vera, and his daughter, after
much thought and research. This was a very difficult
thing for them to do, as they were not entirely sure he
needed to be in a facility. They made the decision to
admit him because they were afraid for him and could
see no way to keep him at home.

Besides his memory loss, he was unable to
make himself clear to strangers, as he had a condition
called "expressive aphasia." Not that he was clear with
his family, but through familiarity they could
frequently guess what he wanted. Also, Tom had
begun wandering. When he wandered away from
home, even though they lived in the country, Vera was
afraid he was going to go out one day and not be able
to get back. She spent many an anxious hour in the
car searching for Tom, and thankfully always found

him. Tom's wife and daughter were in a quandary because, besides his memory and speech problems, Tom could still dress and feed himself, get to the toilet and read the paper. Vera was not sure he understood what he read, but he spent the morning, as he had for forty years, reading the paper.

Tom was 6'4" and thin to the point of being bony, with the rangy strength of a man who had spent much of his life out-of-doors. He would often go out without a coat, and if he did get lost, Vera was fearful he would suffer hypothermia.

In an effort to minimize mistakes, Vera determined to learn all she could about Tom's disease. She immersed herself in every resource available in her community. By the time she brought Tom to our facility, she was convinced that it was the best place for him to be safe.

Once he was living in a community, he was easily redirected, pleasant and extremely gentlemanly, holding doors for those people less physically capable than he. Though relatively non-verbal, he would point at things he wanted, could feed himself, ate well, and took his medications without difficulty.

One day, Tom was walking in the hall when he suddenly knelt down on both knees and appeared to be looking for something. Tom experienced some level of difficulty in getting up again, and as the nurse, I was concerned about his falling, even from a kneeling position, not to mention the rug burns he might get from kneeling on carpet for an extended period of time.

I called his daughter to see if she could shed light on what he was doing, but she too was stumped. "Did he garden? What did he do for work or recreation?" I tried to think of all the questions to ask, but nothing I suggested triggered her memory.

Tom had not been a gardener, and for work he had gone to an office. Even though their home was on a large amount of acreage, he did not do much with it, besides mow the grass. Tom had liked big equipment and had only given up his riding mower after he had flattened a bed of Vera's flowers in error. Though Tom loved the out-of-doors, he was not much of a hunter. He had liked fishing, but his behavior did not match up with anything we could think of. His daughter promised to check with the rest of the family and call me back.

When she did, she told me her brother had provided the answer. When they were children, Tom had raised baby chicks every spring. The chicks were kept in an incubator in the barn, and because the incubator was built low to the ground, Tom had to get down on his knees to see how the chicks were doing. He had given this up years ago, which is why no one thought about the chicks.

His daughter brought in a low, short bench with a 2" lip all the way around. We kept it in his room, and filled it with stuffed baby chicks and put a brightly colored top on stilts, over the table. Tom would sit in a chair by the hour and watch the chicks. Thankfully he stopped kneeling in the hallways. This adjustment only satisfied Tom for a couple of months. After that he ignored the bench in his room altogether, but thankfully never went back to kneeling down in the hall.

Frequently, it is a mystery as to what someone with Alzheimer's is thinking or doing and if they cannot express themselves it can be impossible to figure out. Asking people with dementia questions can be an exercise in frustration and futility for everyone concerned. Family can be a great help in plumbing what a given person may think. Hopefully, together they can get it figured out. Individuals with this disease cannot stay with an idea, so solutions may be temporary. That is both a blessing and a curse. The goal should always be to give the person with dementia some respite from their anxiety, along with some joy, remembering, all the while, that all they have, and are capable of, are moments of delight.

Chapter Twenty-three

GROOMING

Grooming is a concern for people with dementia because staying clean and dry can avoid other health concerns, like skin breakdown.

Bathing should be done when someone is dirty, and on a regular basis, but probably not more than twice per week. To bathe them more frequently can create problems, because their skin is both thin and dry, and therefore susceptible to abrasion.

Using Peri-Wash (a commercial product found in any drug store and specifically made for frequent use on the delicate tissue of the anal area), and hand washing after using the toilet are the two critically important issues. People with dementia may lose awareness of when they have a bowel movement and can wipe themselves improperly. It is very important that this function be monitored for obvious reasons.

Grooming covers both areas of preparing to be dressed, and getting ready for bed. Though I touch generally on grooming in some other chapters, it should be stated here that it is of primary importance to keep the person with dementia clean. They will feel better, even though the intellectual process and the reasons for keeping clean are forgotten.

Shaving males can be dangerous and switching to an electric razor a problem. Sometimes they can do this function on their own, but eventually they will require help.

As part of an older person's grooming, there are issues of eye glasses and hearing aids. A person with dementia may not be able to advise anyone that they cannot hear. They cannot tell caregivers that their hearing aid battery is failing or dead, so the caregiver needs to anticipate this and change the batteries regularly. The batteries should be changed once a week for hearing aids to work effectively, and a ready supply of batteries should be kept on hand.

Glasses can be kept next to the bed, preferably in a case, though some people like to wear them around their neck on a chain. An eye exam, while important to a person who is cognizant, is useless for an individual with dementia. If a person is squinting, have the family buy the next strongest glasses at the pharmacy.

As the person's dementia progresses, families may want to remove glasses, hearing aids, and false teeth from access by the individual. These items may be given to the person at the end of their grooming routine, but not left for the person to remember. Individuals with dementia may get to a point where all these items become more annoying than helpful. Frequently, persons with advanced dementia will throw them away, wrapped in tissue, or hide the items in illogical places. Then, of course, they do not remember where the items are.

Personal care is very important to each person's well being, and needs to be monitored so that issues do not arise without appropriate warning. If this happens, then an intervention can be put in place to fix the problem.

Families or caregivers need to ask the person, "Will you let me help you with that?" Sometimes the person with dementia will refuse, saying, "I can do it myself," and often they can. But keep asking, because there will come a time when they cannot.

Help with grooming is necessary because individuals with dementia not only forget how to do a task, but why they do the task. Left to their own devices, grooming can cease altogether. A lack of grooming can be a hallmark of dementia's onset

Taking physical care of someone with dementia can be very difficult. Families usually do not want to take the person's independence away, much less their dignity. Professional caregivers are trained to interact with a person who has dementia. Families need to realize that caring for someone with dementia is not a one-person job, no matter how much they love the person.

Chapter Twenty-four

FINGERNAILS

The fingernails of people with dementia need to be filed regularly and that filing can be done by anyone. Cutting is an issue, because like toenails, if nails are hard or brittle and a caregiver cuts the person's skin, that then becomes a problem. Any piercing of the skin is considered surgery and beyond a caregiver's scope of practice. Family members are allowed to cut the fingernails of a person with dementia—but are not allowed to delegate this responsibility. Of course, they can cut someone as easily as the next person, but family is privileged. Unlike toenails, which can be addressed by a podiatrist, the family needs to decide who takes care of this procedure, and what should be done about fingernails.

Every time hands are washed, someone needs to clean under the fingernails. The underneath part of fingernails can be a hotbed of infection if left unattended. Soft plastic nail scrubbers can be used effectively. Individuals with dementia can get feces under their nails just by wiping themselves incorrectly.

Because their skin is thin and dry, most elders scratching an itch can cause problems, like breaks in the surface of the skin. This can lead to the more serious issues of skin infections, skin tears, or even cellulitis. Cellulitis is an infection of the dermal layer of the skin which can require the taking of an antibiotic to effect a cure, and left untreated it can lead to hospitalization. Something as simple as a fragrance-free lotion applied to the extremities twice daily can help avoid problems, as less dryness means less itching, and less scratching.

Many women have had manicures over their lifetime and it is an enjoyable process for them. A problem arises if they want to wear their nails long. Family can be very useful in talking these ladies into shorter nails, whether or not they are covered with polish. Obviously, naked nails are preferable because they allow caregivers to see if the nails need cleaning.

Most men, on the other hand, have not had manicures, and some balk at the idea. Where some men are concerned one is more likely to get the response, "I can do it myself!" These men must be approached differently, but again family members can be helpful in this area. Even if a man cuts himself with a jagged fingernail, he will often have the attitude that it is no big deal and does not require cleaning or a band-aid. However, it does require cleaning at this age, and in this instance a nurse can be helpful. The current geriatric generation still responds positively to authority, and if the nurse says it must be addressed, so be it!

As dementia progresses, things like cleaning fingernails and hand washing become even more important. Partially this is true because the person's sense of smell changes and partially because they lose intellectual process. People with dementia fail to understand why touching feces is a problem. Like little children, if they are uncomfortable they will dig out matter, or put feces in places that are inappropriate, like a trash basket.

The use of a nail brush to keep the area under fingernails, cleaner than hand washing alone and is highly recommended.

Caregivers need to remember to be careful when handling body fluids, even if the person has dementia.

Avoiding infection by washing hands and keeping fingernails clean and short, can go a long way to keeping someone with dementia safe.

Chapter Twenty-five

TOENAIL FUNGUS

Somewhere around fifty percent of all elderly have some type of toenail fungus. Getting onychomycosis is not a reflection of being dirty, or of improper foot care —it is bad luck. There are three kinds of this fungus and depending on the type contracted, the nails may turn yellow, gray, brown or black. The nail may become brittle or crack and it may separate from the skin or nail bed. Secondary infections are also possible if bacteria get into an open area in the skin of the foot.

Basically there are three varieties of onychomycosis —DSO, WSO or PSO. Once one toenail is infected, the fungus can and often does, spread to the other toes. While over-the-counter products can curb or possibly control the progress, there is no cure for the problem. Even an oral prescription medication may not be the answer, as frequently the fungus will return, months after a course of treatment is completed. A second problem with the oral prescription medication is that it can be hard on the liver (already slowed in function by age), and liver studies must be done while taking this medication. There are in excess of fifteen pages of treatments on the internet for fungal toenails, and none of them can promise a cure. Everything from tea tree oil to Vicks VapoRub to Listerine has been touted as an aid by someone. Some of these possibly help in some cases, but their effectiveness is not, however, universal. Several companies have laser treatments in trials to obtain FDA approval to treat toenail fungus, but those processes are still pending. Once the process is approved by the FDA, it will probably be expensive, at least for a while.

A visit to the podiatrist to have these nails cut and monitored is a good idea. If your loved one has diabetes, it can be critically important. Diabetic foot care is essential to your loved one's health. Of course, family can cut and file the toenails themselves, but if a family member flinches or moves suddenly and skin is cut, it has the potential to cause critical complications. In most states, Medicare will pay to have a podiatrist cut fungal toenails, even if you have to transport your loved one to an office.

Caregivers and even nurses cannot perform this service because if they happen, however inadvertently, to cut someone's skin in the process of trimming their toenails, they have technically performed surgery, which is out of their scope of practice.

Fungal toenails need care and should not be ignored. As a student nurse I watched an operation to replace a gentleman's hip. The man had been wheelchair bound due to his hip degeneration. When he was put on the operating table his toenails, all ten of them, had grown so long they were curled over the ends of his toes. Even if he had been able to walk with his hip, he would have been unable to walk because of the lack of care of his fungal toenails.

Fungal nails, whether they occur on the foot or the hand, should be under the care of an M.D., and your loved one's primary care physician can refer to a podiatrist for foot care, and a dermatologist for hand care. Whatever he or she decides is the best way to effectively change the problem.

Whatever you do, do not ignore fungal toenails.

Chapter Twenty-six

TEETH

Whether a person has their own teeth or dentures, once they develop dementia, the care of their teeth requires addressing by their primary caregiver. Unless an electric tooth brush is frightening to the person with dementia, it is easier to handle for someone else who may be cleaning their teeth, and may be able to do a more thorough job. If the person has never used an electric toothbrush, now in the early dementia stages, may be the time to introduce it.

Routine makes most people with dementia feel more secure, and frequently, even though it is difficult to learn something new, they can be conditioned to a new routine. Regular tooth care can avoid a lot of other health problems, but whether or not a family member is kept at home or placed in a community, they should have a dentist. If your family dentist is willing to take on, or continue with, the dental care of a person dementia, that is ideal. Otherwise, as your loved one's advocate, you need to call the local dental offices to find out who is willing to take on dementia patients. Many dentists do not specialize in dementia patients, or they have practices which make caring for a person with dementia difficult. Some dental hygienists have a practice where they will come to your home or living facility and take care of cleaning the person's teeth. These practitioners are generally good with dementia patients, and often much of their practice is made up of such a group. The advantages are obvious: your love one gets good care, and a hygienist can alert you to potential problems that would require a dental visit.

Remember, with age tissue losses tensile strength. This is also true of a person's gums—they eventually recede, even if tooth and gum care has been good. Due to gum recession, dentures deteriorate to a juncture where they do not fit. Once this happens, dentures can cause sores. Frequently, a person with dementia will hide dentures. He or she does not want to wear them because they are annoying or hurt, and the person has lost the ability to reason out what the benefits may be. If this happens, it will happen in the later stages of dementia, but being aware is forearmed.

While a loved one is capable, and if they still have their own teeth, flossing is of paramount importance, both to keep the teeth clean and to minimize gum recession. Unfortunately, there is no way to determine exactly when a person with dementia can still floss and when that ability is lost, until it happens. If you or a caregiver is having difficulty getting someone to floss, it may be time to reassess this particular skill. There is a product on the market which is a piece of floss stretched between two ends of a plastic loop, which is effective as a flossing agent. Be aware that the other end of the item is a tooth pick which can be dangerous, not just because it is sharp, but also because individuals with dementia may not experience pain in the same way we do and may do something inappropriate if allowed to manipulate the floss/toothpick item while alone. This item must be locked away when not in use.

A caregiver will need to help with the chore of flossing, while being careful of the bite reflex. If this is triggered, the person will bite down regardless of what may be in the way, like a finger. The person is not aware that they have bitten down and may need several verbal prompts of open their mouth.

Daily soaking of dentures overnight using a commercial denture cleaner in a cup of water is recommended. Never brush dentures with a tooth brush, as over time it will take off the finish. Some individuals, usually women, in the early part of their dementia will not be seen without their teeth. Soaking dentures overnight is ideal, but even soaking for an hour while one gets ready for bed is better than nothing. The dentures can then be rinsed, dried with a soft cloth and returned to the person's mouth. Denture cleaning material needs only to be available when a caregiver is present to monitor its use.

If a person loses a tooth, you may want to consider where it is and whether or not it will interfere with the person's eating ability, if it is not replaced. Again remember, that a person with dementia has a hard time sitting still for any kind of procedure, as well as an inability to follow directions.

Teeth, and their good care, are crucial to a person's health. If the person has their own teeth, many problems can be avoided, health increased, and potential pain decreased.

Chapter Twenty-seven

PHONE SERVICE: LOUIS' STORY

Families are frequently in a quandary when it comes to phone service. If the person with dementia can still use a phone, it can be programmed to call family members only. This can be done with pictures next to the phone buttons, but it does not affect incoming phone calls from control systems that continuously dial numbers until they get an answer. The people on the other end do not really care if they are talking to an elderly person or one with Alzheimer's—they do not care if the number is on a "no call list." They only care that a person to commits to taking whatever they are offering. They will ask for a credit card number over the phone, and sometimes try to send items C.O.D. Most facilities will refuse this type of solicitation. The problem is, an unlisted phone number does not stop people with the intention of putting over a scam.

Louis was a short man, near 5'6" with a full head of silver hair, a winning smile, and was looked upon as a dapper dresser. He always wore a dress shirt and one of his rather extensive collections of vests. Louis had lived in an assisted-living community for more than five years. The decision, made by his family, for Louis to stay in the assisted living community, was because Louis had begun to lose decision-making capabilities, even though he continued to be upbeat and cheerful. He could even still play cards, after a fashion.

Louis had a very attentive daughter, Marie, who had his Power of Attorney. That daughter lived close and often made an effort to come visit, take him out to family functions, and phone him on a weekly basis.

One day Louis came down to the desk and announced he had won two million dollars. Appropriately enough, we congratulated him and asked if we could help with the paperwork. He said that he had come to tell us because he needed one of us to drive him to the bank where he intended to withdraw $5,000 and take it to a gentleman who would meet him outside the local Dollar Store. This man was to meet Louis in the parking lot and would give him two million dollars in exchange for Louis' $5,000. Louis said there was no paper work necessary, as the gentleman had called him on his phone.

We immediately notified Marie (the Power of Attorney) . At her behest, the State Attorney General used Louis' information to set up a sting operation. Meanwhile Marie arrived and carefully told him that the offer had been a scam, at which point he replied, "I hope the cops get him and put him away—that is a terrible thing to try to fool old people!" Though he wanted to believe he had won two million dollars, luckily he was still in a condition where he readily believed his daughter.

Be diligent about the phone. Try to convince your parents that they do not need their own phone. Tell them you will call them each day, and the facility will alert them when a call comes. They may not remember the time, but they will remember you said you would call. You don't need the added stress of your loved one calling the police in the middle of the night, as one woman did. On the phone they may sound like they know what they are talking about, but they do not. When your loved one gets to a point where mistakes with the phone are being made, it is time to remove the phone.

Remember, all people with dementia will lose ability over time. Unfortunately there does not exist a predictable time table. For instance, one cannot say that they will lose the phone ability in their third year. There is a fine line between encouraging their independence, keeping them safe and controlling paranoid reactions.

Chapter Twenty-eight

SKIN INTEGRITY

When we are young, our skin is attached to the tissue underneath (the dermis). As we age, our skin loosens and loses tensile strength. The tissue appears to separate from the dermis and we end up with the "flobbys," that tissue which wiggles on the back side of our upper arms or on our thighs. It is also why we are subject to skin tears. Unfortunately no amount of exercise, eating a balanced diet, the use of lotion or anything else we do makes much of a difference. Excess weight exacerbates all the problems anyone may have, but it really doesn't effect our getting the flobbys.

Beyond the fact that our skin becomes thinner, as age increases, it also becomes dryer, slides on the dermis, tears more easily, and is difficult to manage in the healing process. Skin tears can be small or large.

There are several steps one needs to take to help skin tears heal. 1) Stop the bleeding with pressure. This is not a quick process and often takes between five or ten minutes of applied pressure. Skin tears look awful, and can get infected if they are not taken care of properly, but, generally, they are not serious in and of themselves. 2) Clean the area with normal saline (available as "Wound Wash" by Blairex), or an alternative is a good commercial cleanser that will cleanse the wound and not sting the patient. When cleaning a wounded area, one needs to pat at the tear gently, so that bleeding does not restart. 3) Next, assess the size and how jagged the edges of the wound appear. Steri-strips can be applied, and the wound then covered with a Tegaderm—a thin sterile dressing (all available in any drug store). If the cut is large, or very jagged, a piece of PolyMem can be used to protect the wound, and which can then be covered by a Tegaderm. Each of these items, as well as 4 x 4 gauze (sponges), are available in most drug stores and should be kept in stock, in your first aid kit. If infection is a possibility, often determined by what caused the cut in the first place, a thin layer of antibiotic ointment can be applied with a Q-tip to the side of the PolyMem that goes on the wound. If a wound is big enough, it may require stitches and probably should be assessed by an M.D.

The follow-up to a skin tear treatment is also important. Though a dressing may technically stay on the tear for seven days, it should be checked every three days for signs and symptoms of infection, which include redness, swelling, heat, pain, and discharge of pus. A skin tear may seep sero-sanguineous fluid, which, if allowed to collect, can grow bacteria. Therefore, changing the dressing every three days until healing starts to take place is not a bad idea. If used alone for a smaller tear, steri-strips can be left in place until they fall off by themselves, because the wound is healing and can be assessed with the strips in place, or through the Tegaderm.

Recently, MRSA, both in and out of hospitals, has been in the news. MRSA stands for "methacillian resistant staphylococcus aureus," which is a bacterium that causes difficult-to-treat infections in humans. Although staph aureus is always on our skin, as the body's largest organ, the skin protects us from all types of staph, which could lead to dangerous infections if allowed to penetrate the skin. The use of universal precautions and hand washing can control how staph gets spread around. MRSA is only a more dangerous form of staph because it is not vulnerable to ordinary broad spectrum antibiotics, but if caregivers are careful and use universal precautions, MRSA can be avoided like any other bacteria.

There are two other skin conditions which are frequently a problem in the elderly population: seborrheic dermatitis (known in infants as cradle cap), and dry skin. The best way to deal with all problems is prevention. When the skin is not cleaned and moisturized frequently enough it becomes dry and can flake off, tear or split. The thin skin of the elderly is more vulnerable to this process.

Because their skin is thin, and since this population rarely does anything that would make them get dirty, bathing should ideally be done only twice per week, unless treating a specific problem, and then the doctor's instructions need to be followed.

For some reason, individuals with dementia frequently do not want anyone to touch their hair, or they may even fear getting their heads wet. If this comes up, try a trip to the beauty salon for women, or for men, the barber. I have witnessed women who will not wait five minutes for anything else, sit quietly for more than an hour awaiting their turn at the hairdresser. If a person with dementia will let a caregiver wash his hair, it is a good idea to use baby shampoo with a "no tears" formula. This does not need to be done more than once per week. What is important is stimulating the scalp by scrubbing to avoid dry skin build up.

Moisturizer is hugely important and should be put on the hands and other extremities at least twice daily. Perfumed lotions can be problematic due to allergies. The lotion should be non-allergic and in an easily used dispenser. Moisturized skin is more resistant to most skin problems. Once skin is dry and cracking, it opens the person up to a myriad of problems, not the least of which is discomfort.

Keep in mind that as dementia progresses a loved one may not be able to tell us that they are uncomfortable, or even itchy; instead might act out, or rub (scratch) a spot raw. Caregivers need to be alert for all skin changes, and those changes must be addressed in a timely manner.

Chapter Twenty-nine

HALLUCINATIONS: GRACE'S STORY

When Alice and her husband moved to the country from the city, they brought along Alice's mother, Grace, with them. Grace was eighty-six and could still drive, though she had given up her car before they moved. Grace felt because she did not know the streets, she would be better off relying on cabs, or her daughter.

Grace's balance was excellent; she had been a dancer, and she walked independently with no physical aids. Many of her friends thought she was a marvel to be so flexible at her advanced age.

What Grace wanted most when she moved to town was an apartment with a view of the bay. Grace was also adamant about not wanting to live with Alice and her husband. Besides not wanting to feel like a burden, Grace wished to be independent, a theme expressed both before and after her husband died.

Unfortunately, after only a year had passed since her move, hallucinations began. Fortunately, they were benign hallucinations. She would call up Alice to have her come over and see the mermaids in the bay. It did not occur to Grace that the presence of mermaids was exceptional in and of itself.

Except for those late afternoon hallucinations, Grace appeared to be functioning at much the same level that she always had. Then, without a trauma, the hallucinations became worse and her family, realizing that something was very different, requested she be admitted to a geri-psych unit in the city, several hours from the town in which they all lived. The physicians there tried several medications but the side effects were worse than whatever help the drug was supposed to be. Grace complained of leg pains and said that her legs felt like jelly. So she was taken off all medication. The physicians diagnosed her with dementia of the Alzheimer's type, with hallucinations. Though Grace returned to her condominium, Alice knew she was not safe there. But, before Alice could find an appropriate dementia community, Grace went out for a walk, fell, broke her collarbone and was admitted to the local hospital.

When Grace moved into an "assisted living for memory care" unit, she said she felt she was still independent, though due to the collarbone break, she was using a walker to steady her gait. She was still having some hallucinations, but they were neither frequent nor frightening to her.

Grace's two largest issues were that she would not lie down in a bed and her legs were scaling. She also had a history of some mild ankle edema and was on a mild blood pressure medication. The bed problem was solved by Alice, who bought her mother a couch. The scaling leg problem was also addressed by Alice, who came to the community every day to soak her mother's legs, dry them, remove the lose scale by brisk rubbing with a dry towel, and applying lotion to her legs and feet. This first-aid worked, and the problem of scaly legs cleared up, though Grace continued to receive lotion to her legs twice a day as a preventative measure.

Grace also had a hearing problem and had worn hearing aides for a while. Eventually, she began misplacing them or would refuse to wear them. She would tell the caregiver helping her, "those aren't mine, they belong to my roommate." No one was ever able to determine if this was an excuse or another hallucination, as there was no roommate. Grace also used this excuse anytime she didn't want to do something a caregiver requested, like brushing her hair or teeth. "That", she would chirp, pointing to an item, "belongs to my roommate and she would be angry if I used it." While she was in the psychiatric facility, Grace had a roommate, but that was the only time. Alzheimer's patients usually have good historical memory, but poor current memory; however this is a generality and not true in all cases.

Feeling her mother would want to have a conversation despite a lack of hearing aids, Alice bought her mother a pocket talker, which is an over-the-counter device one uses by putting a tiny earpiece in the ear, turning the device on, and listening, as the unit is controlled by the talker. Alice found this tool helpful for about three months, during which time the most useful thing she learned was to not argue with Grace. Whatever her mother said she accepted as valid, and she found it more fun and easier than trying to reorient her mother to reality. Remember that denying someone's reality, be it a dementia patient or a child, is an exercise in futility. The person who tells you the tale believes it is the truth.

As time went on, however, Grace did start to decline and began falling asleep in odd places. She was not participating in activities, partially because they were beyond her, and partially because her hearing was so poor. The community managers met with the family to discuss moving Grace to a higher level of care where she would get more hands-on physical care and attention-appropriate activities. The family agreed and she was moved. Grace enjoyed her new activities and engaged in them more frequently because they were appropriate for her stage of dementia.

Then Grace had a fall. She was taken to ER immediately, but the x-rays were negative, and she was returned to the community. Upon her arrival Grace began to complain of pain, refused to walk, and would only sit in a wheelchair most of the time. It should be noted that pain is one of the first things to rule out when a person with dementia acts out or behaves differently from their norm. Pain, thirst, the need to urinate or evacuate, the need for food and the need for sleep, are all triggers for some form of agitated behavior.

Grace was given pain medication, and assessed for hospice. She had quit eating and was only minimally drinking. Hospice gave her really strong pain medication and took her off all other medications. There were days when Grace would not get out of bed, and most everyone, including Alice, thought that the end was near.

Still, Alice was bothered by what she was seeing. She really knew her mother well. She had been a participant in her mother's life both before and during her decline into dementia. Alice felt there was something more wrong, something that the physicians were missing. Alice insisted on getting Grace an MRI and it showed what the x-rays had missed: compression fractures. Alice's mother went through a vertebroplasty and her pain immediately resolved. Grace actually started eating again and graduated from hospice. Once she was back on a regular routine, Alice thought she experienced her mother as more alert and responsive, and believed it was because she was receiving no medications. Alice took Grace to see her primary care physician and Grace was not put back on anything but a daily 81mg. aspirin.

Today Grace lives happily at the dementia community. She engages in activities and enjoys visits from her family. Recently Alice came to visit. Not finding her mother at her regular place, she was about to ask where her mother might be when from across the main room she heard her mother call, "Yoo-hoo, I'm right over here!" Grace had recognized Alice.

There are several lessons to be learned from this story. First, always pay attention to pain, whether or not it can be verbalized. Keep going if you feel something is wrong. If Alice had not insisted on further testing what would have been the result? The elderly cannot advocate for themselves. As their children we must advocate for them. Second, have all medications reviewed at least once per year and see if the physician is willing to allow the patient a "drug holiday," a time without drugs to see what happens. Family must do their part to observe closely, report accurate findings to the physician, and put the person back on a given medication if the physician recommends it. Sometimes, though, after a person begins receiving a drug, over time their body changes and it may no longer be appropriate. Unless someone is watching, the person just keeps on taking the drug. The third, Grace was just lucky!

When Grace had her moment of clarity, it was a gift!

Chapter Thirty

INCONTINENCE

Incontinence is one of the most difficult aspects of dementia for families to acknowledge, and certainly one of the most difficult for patients to deal with, until their dementia progresses and wearing pull-ups becomes the norm. From the time we are very young, we are trained to use the toilet. It feels somehow degrading to lose bladder control, especially for men.

Most women who have had a least one full term pregnancy are to some degree incontinent of urine. It is called "stress incontinence" and generally comes from a loosening of the pelvic floor muscles so that when someone is coughing, laughing, running or lifting, leakage may occur. Women also produce less estrogen as a result of aging, so some loss of urine may be due to a flaccid bladder, and produce overflow incontinence. These are both normal kinds of incontinence and can be mitigated by doing exercises of the pelvic floor muscles called *Kegel exercises* several times a day.

Whatever the reason for incontinence, family is often embarrassed by its presence. Caregivers and nurses who are familiar with the elderly deal with the situation all the time. Rest assured, incontinence is the rule more than the exception.

Urge incontinence is the feeling that one needs to urinate frequently. There are medications that can arrest or improve this temporarily, but, when taking any medication, one must be aware that there are side effects. Even though a medication is designed to do a particular job, it must work with the person's body. It may work for a while then not be as much help as it was in the beginning. Sometimes the side effects can be worse than the problem. This is not to say the medicine does not work or that the physician who prescribed it was remiss in doing so, it simply was not effective for that person. If a person has more than one type of incontinence at the same time, the problem may be confused, and medication will not work properly.

At the care facility where I worked, a resident named Elizabeth had two sons. One son, Richard, was very realistic about this mother's condition, and the other son, George, was not. George kept thinking Elizabeth would get better.

When Elizabeth moved into an assisted living facility, she was incontinent and wore pads. As Elizabeth's disease progressed, her incontinence worsened and she began to soil her underwear. Our recommendation was for Elizabeth to begin wearing pull-ups, but George wouldn't hear of it. He prevailed on her M.D. to give his mother medication. Elizabeth took the medication, but endured several side effects, among them dry mouth, insomnia, and urinary retention. It made almost no difference in Elizabeth's incontinence. Finally the M.D. talked to Elizabeth and together they made the decision to take her off the medication, particularly because the beneficial effects were minimal and the side effects were affecting Elizabeth's quality of life.

George had a fit. He did not want his mother to be incontinent. He did not want to do her urine saturated laundry. It was clearly George's problem, not his mother's.

While some people can stay clean by wearing panty liners, others have a higher level of incontinence and require pants (pull-ups) that can absorb urine and the odor. In the early stages of dementia, individuals may frequently have a really hard time emotionally, accepting that they are incontinent. Besides the fact that incontinence can be a sign of old age, individuals sometimes feel it is a sign that they can no longer control their body functions, and those feelings make them resistant to help. Help, however, is out there, and one of the most effective ways to aid this situation is through instituting a toileting schedule, both to void and defecate at certain times of the day. This helps to avoid accidents.

Frequently a person will not tell family members that they have this issue, and it comes as a shock when the person moves into a community and the nursing staff advises the family of the problem. Staff does not want the family to solve the problem, but the family may need to talk to their loved one to make the process of receiving more help acceptable. After all, patients have not wet their pants since they were babies. Being empathetic about this issue is paramount both to the patient and their family members. Family members can feel it is inappropriate or embarrassing for their loved one to have this issue. That, of course, is the family reacting to how the person used to be, not how they are now. If the family treats the condition as no big deal, the person will often follow suit.

The issues that arise around incontinence are skin breakdown and skin irritation. When changing someone with dementia, aloe-vera gel can be applied to the skin. It is both cooling and healing and can even be applied to the vaginal areas with ease by placing some gel on a tissue. The gel is great to clean someone up. If the irritation is more serious of if the bowel is involved, a barrier cream may need to be applied every time someone goes to the toilet to avoid ulcers and heal minor skin lesions. Older individuals are at risk, however, and should be checked regularly, whether at home or in assisted living. Incontinence is a problem, but it can be addressed positively and the person with the problem can be helped to feel "okay" about it.

Fecal incontinence does not usually come up until the person is in late Stage 6 or 7; in other words, near the end of life. Sometimes a person never becomes incontinent of feces. If they do, it is important to understand that the anal sphincter can lose its ability to feel, so that the person having the bowel movement does not realize they are defecating.

By the time fecal incontinence is a problem, the individual is generally wearing pull-ups or some other form of diaper. A bowel program, encouraging the person to evacuate at the same time every day, can minimize accidents. This type of program is recommended even in the early stages of dementia in order to help avoid messy problems in the future.

Chapter Thirty-one

BACTERIA

Bacteria smell when they are exposed to oxygen. When you become aware of an odor, whether it is from the body, the mouth, the feet or a smell in a room, you can be reasonably sure it is either bacteria or mold—if you live in a location where it can grow.

Deodorant is appropriate to use if a person has a naturally strong body odor, but do not use an antiperspirant on older people. Be sure you read the label on any underarm product you consider buying to ensure it does not contain antiperspirant. Many commercial products that advertise as deodorants actually do contain antiperspirants. The chemicals in antiperspirants contain ingredients designed to retard perspiration. Most elderly have problems regulating body temperature as it is, and most of them are not doing the kind of physical activity that would make them perspire. Since perspiration is the body's natural way of cooling itself, products that slow or stop this process can be harmful and lead to dehydration—a huge problem in the elderly.

Urine is sterile as it leaves the body, but it picks up bacteria as it passes over the skin. If there is an odor emanating from the urine itself, there is every possibility that an infection of some kind is present, be it yeast or bacterial. If you smell urine in a room, chances are that someone or something is wet, and has been wet for a while. The person who has had the accident does not know or cannot remember what he or she did. It is the responsibility of the caregivers to find and fix the problem. If your loved one is living in a care home and has had an accident, tell someone in authority. Often people in the early stages of dementia will realize they have wet themselves, and will attempt to wash or dry their pants in inappropriate ways.

A smell does not have to come from urine or feces. A family member came to me one day saying that her father's feet were not clean. When she had changed his socks to go out, multiple skin cells came off with the old socks and the feet stank. After investigating the situation, it was determined that this gentleman refused to allow anyone to touch his feet. Apparently he had always been this way and it became exaggerated when he got dementia. Even though he was being showered twice a week by caregivers, he would refuse to allow anyone to wash his feet. He said he would do it himself. In an effort to help someone maintain their independence, caregivers are taught to allow a person with dementia to do what they can for themselves. After discussion with the family, they bought him a foot spa. His daughter then gave him three spas with caregivers present to normalize the process. Eventually this gentleman would allow caregivers to soak his feet, dry them off, and apply lotion. The dirty foot problem was solved!

This brings up a very important point. Because an individual moves into a community does not mean that they will automatically get perfect care. This is not a one person job. Family members, and the things they notice, are a community's number one resource when it comes to making changes or solving problems brought to their attention. Of course caregivers try to catch everything, but the person still trusts family most and will share with them things they will not, or cannot, tell a caregiver.

If someone has an odor, investigate it. There is a cause and it probably can be fixed.

Chapter Thirty-two

CHANGING ROLES: SARA'S STORY

Sara, a woman whose mother, Olive, had died of Alzheimer's, told me something I found both interesting and profound.

"The hardest thing I had to accept, and it took time to work it out," she said, "was the difficulty in the reversal of roles between Mom and myself. Role reversal is extremely difficult. All your life you have been used to getting sage advice from a person, then this cloud comes over, and the person you have known all this time, disappears. It is devastating."

I found this fascinating, because it made me think that for everyone, some shift, be it major or minor, is what gets to be difficult and becomes the issue that requires work. It is where we, as individuals, have to stretch. Profound because it illustrates Sara's truth, and truth is always profound.

When someone gets Alzheimer's disease, or any form of dementia, the process begins slowly and the first item frequently noted by family is a lack of current memory. Someone with dementia may repeat themselves or forget that they visited the doctor last week, but historical memory stays intact for the most part, until much later in the progression. Historical memory is actually held in a different part of the brain than current memory. The reality is, that while family members focus on a loved one's memory loss, thought process is also being affected.

Olive was a caregiving mother in the truest sense of the word. Caregiving to her children, husband or anyone in need, came naturally to her. Olive loved helping, taking care of everyone within her ken. She had taken care of her parents in their old age; Sara could remember what their life was like having two old, sick people in the house, and the stress it brought. Sara really loved her grandparents and was aware of how difficult their life was, needing the help they did, and feeling that they might be a burden to Olive. Not that Olive ever complained—she did not—but she was certain to obtain long-term care insurance for herself, so that she would not be a burden to Sara and her family in her elder years.

Olive not only took care of her parents, as time went on she took care of her husband, at home. He had Parkinson's, which was followed by a major stroke that left him wheelchair bound along with other functional problems. Sara felt that, over time, the stress of taking care of her Dad for the years she did, added to, if not brought on, her mother's eventual illness. As there is currently no known definitive cause for Alzheimer's, and we do know that stress can exacerbate any illness, Sara may be correct.

Sara was her father's daughter. She was bright, interested in a variety of endeavors, particularly anything scientific, and totally unlike Olive. Sara felt both an aversion and guilt, whenever the issue of personal care came up. Olive had been the perfect caregiver and, like many women of her generation, not only thought that caregiving was an appropriate role for women, but also believed, erroneously, that all women were naturally good at it. Sara wanted to be like her mother, and felt guilty that she was not good at care giving. She was, however, determined to take care of her mother as she had watched her mother take care of her grandparents and father.

It is so difficult, especially when we are young, to see ourselves as having talents separate from those of our parents. Growing up we usually experience our parents as better, smarter, and surer of themselves than we are. We believe, in our hearts, that if our role model is good at something, we should be too. And because we see ourselves in terms of how we think our parents see us, it takes a lot of work to be all right with ourselves as being different from our parents. Added to that is the role model issue. Sons try to emulate their fathers, while girls try to emulate their mothers, and if we fall short, it takes patience, hard work and understanding to get to a place where we are at peace with those differences.

Sara's parents moved into Sara's house as soon as it was purchased, with the idea that Sara and her husband would occupy the ground level, and Sara's parents the basement. As it turned out, though, her father could not use the stairs, so during the move they switched places. Olive loved living on the first floor with the large glass windows and panoramic views.

One of the first indicators of an oncoming change evidenced itself when Olive thought she had always lived in Sara's house. Then, when Sara's father died suddenly, it was a blow to everyone, but especially to Olive. She had been operating under the illusion that because she took such good care of her husband, and refused to put him in a nursing home, he would go on indefinitely. As often happens, one tragedy follows another, and Olive's brother died three months later.

Sara remembered that shortly after her father's death, her mother began to decline. One incident that stuck with Sara was that Olive had been a stickler for folding and putting away the laundry in a very specific manner. Sara noticed that her mother was still putting the laundry away, but folded differently and she was putting it in different places.

Once Olive's brother died, Olive went downhill even faster. Frequently a trauma, like the death of someone close, or sometimes even a minor illness, can trigger an additional decline. Olive began underlining words in magazine ads and when asked what she was doing, replied, "a project for school."

Because her parents had insurance that paid for in-home care, Sara was able to afford live-in help while her father was sick, but she kept it for her mother after her dad died. By this time and with all the odd things that were happening, Sara felt her mother needed someone with her night and day. She was also afraid to leave the house and run errands, or take care of her farm animals, because she might be needed. Even though someone was there all the time, Sara was trapped in a caregiver nightmare; torn between what she needed to do, and afraid to leave the house.

As last straws often do, they happen when they are least expected, and always at night. Sara woke up because she heard what sounded like water dripping in the closet. She got out of bed to check and to her dismay she found water coming through the ceiling around the light fixture. Sara raced upstairs to find Olive in the bathroom, the one above Sara's closet, with about two inches of water on the floor. Olive was standing in the water with a totally bewildered expression on her face. The commode had overflowed and Olive just kept flushing, waiting for the water to go down. At that juncture, Sara knew she needed more help for Olive than she or an in-home caregiver could provide.

Sara immediately took her mother to Olive's primary care physician who recommended, and not for the first time, that Sara put her mother in an assisted living community with a focus on memory care, with the idea that the socialization of her peers might be a positive distraction and slow down the disease process.

The physician had tried Olive on the available drugs to mitigate the progression, but the side effects had warranted his stopping those medications. Moving Olive into a dementia facility had the desired effect. Olive was basically a happy person and getting love and care from people who had her best interests at heart, along with visits from her daughter, gave what life she had left quality, serenity and moments of joy.

Sara learned to enjoy Olive as she was, and to let go of the guilt she felt in not being the kind of daughter she thought Olive wanted. At the end, Sara was able to accept Olive's death as she had accepted her life, not without pain, but with peace.

Chapter Thirty-three

WALKING AND FALLS

Sooner or later individuals with dementia will fall. Despite what the professionals do, regardless of the steps one takes to modify individuals' environments, even with 24/7 care, they will fall.

The intention behind providing physical therapy, occupational therapy, modifying the environment, and everyone involved doing their best to keep a loved one safe, is to mitigate the fall, and make it less damaging.

Sometimes families feel that once a loved one is in a community they will be safe and not fall. Untrue. Communities do the same sets of things that you do at home. They remove tripping hazards, pick up throw rugs, keep hallways clear and watch those individuals that are unsteady on their feet. Getting someone to use a walker once they have dementia can be a challenge. I do not say impossible, because some people with dementia take immediately to walkers because they feel safer. Sometimes egos become involved, and they will want to use a cane (or two) that they have been using all along, and these can be dangerous. These aids can also become more confusing to use, as the dementia progresses. Individuals will use the furniture in their apartment or house to move around, and tell you they are fine!

We all know that walking is good exercise. We encourage the elderly, even those who use walkers, to participate in this kind of exercise. The problem arises when someone with dementia becomes fixated on walking and literally will walk till they drop. In the facility in which I worked, we had a lady who did just that, on a walker. We tried to arrange places for her to sit when she got tired, but she would pass them, go twenty feet further and then fall from being exhausted. She could not remember that the chairs were there for her. We arranged for people to be with her frequently, but she would get away and fall. Finally her family hired an outside person just to walk with her, pushing a wheelchair behind her so that when she got tired she had somewhere to sit immediately. One-to-one works well, but every caregiver has to go home at the end of the shift. So having a caregiver to walk with her only worked until she began getting up in the middle of the night, walking with her walker, and falling. Eventually she broke her hip, got put into a wheelchair and that solved her walking problem.

I mention this because problems presented by those with dementia are not simple, often cannot be easily solved, and sometimes cannot be solved at all.

Chapter Thirty-four

WEIGHT AND DIABETES

Excess weight exacerbates every other thing that can go wrong with our bodies. If I had to choose only one thing to tell people in order to maintain reasonably good health, I would tell them to lose weight. The only way to reduce weight, all advertising aside, is to exercise and reduce caloric intake. Obviously it is not the only thing to do, but it is one of the most important.

As we age, our ratio of fat to muscle mass changes. We gain in fat content and lose muscle mass. Women have a greater percentage of change than men, so an exercise routine involving walking, and in general watching one's diet, becomes more important. Despite that fact, as other interests change food can become more important. Eating more fruits and vegetables and less carbohydrates is paramount to good health, along with also eating protein, which is a critical factor in healing.

The time of day one eats also plays a role in how much weight we gain or lose. It is healthier to eat twice daily, instead of three times a day, with the big meal between one and three in the afternoon. This can help one avoid extra, unwanted pounds.

Carrying excess weight makes a person more vulnerable to getting Type II diabetes. Type II reflects one of two processes. Bodies may not make enough insulin or may become insulin resistant. This is an over-simplification of what happens, and I encourage anyone with a diagnosis of Type II diabetes to go to a clinic and learn all they can about this type of diabetes, and why they got this disease. If a person has a first degree relative with diabetes, their chance of getting the disease increases. Most hospitals have diabetes educators who give regular classes to those who need them, at minimal or no cost.

A large percentage of older adults will tell me they are borderline diabetic and control their diabetes with diet. That may be true when a person is able to remember what is done or not, or what is eaten and what they must be careful about. A person with dementia will not remember the rules. A diet must be prescribed by an M.D. or dietician, and followed meticulously in order to work.

The family of a woman at our facility provided the community dietician with a menu and a complete list of things the woman could eat. To add to her diabetic problems, she was extremely dairy sensitive, and if she ate dairy, she got diarrhea. Given the opportunity, however, she would eat real ice cream. She had a niece who came a far distance to see her, so her visits were not frequent. When she did visit, the niece would take the woman out to buy her a milk shake. Naturally, being diabetic and dairy sensitive, the woman would get sick. We tried explaining to the niece about the problem, to no avail. Eventually the woman's daughter had to restrict the niece's visits because the niece thought we were being mean to the woman by depriving her of the things she loved to eat. It was interesting that the niece in question was overweight, herself.

Part of the difficulty of following a diet is that people want to eat when they get bored, and people with dementia have very short attention spans. Despite activities designed to stimulate them, they revert to eating easily.

Eating is also a social activity and people with dementia crave the attention they get at a table with other people. It is inconsequential whether it is in a community or at home. Sometimes people in the early stages of dementia will sit at a table, just waiting for someone's presence.

Chapter Thirty-five

TRAVELING

For someone with dementia, travel can be an overwhelming experience. Routine and sameness are the things that make a person without dementia bored, and a person with dementia feel safe, even if the person loved to travel once upon a time.

Up until a person has progressed to Stage 4, travel is a possibility, depending upon the individual person. First of all, they have to want to go. Be sure to ask several times, because they can forget what they decided or said about the subject. If you are getting a mixed message it is probably better to cancel the trip.

The second thing to be sure of, is that the person who wants your loved one to visit needs is aware of the need to pick them up. They are not capable of getting their luggage alone and meeting a vehicle at curbside. They will not be able to recognize a particular vehicle. It is a little like having a five year old travel alone.

If a trip is necessary and you cannot accompany your loved one, there are several things you must do:

- Contact the designated airline and advise them you are sending a person on their airline who has some dementia and that this person must be escorted to the designated contact person in the luggage area—a person who will be responsible for the loved one from there. You must make sure that your loved one is capable of staying in their designated airline seat and not wander around the plane. If you are not sure if this is possible, your loved one must be accompanied in flight.

- If the person who is flying needs to go to the restroom, the flight attendant needs to accompany them and wait for them, unless you can assure the airline that the person can perform this function alone. The airline attendant needs to caution the person not to lock the door, unless there is a way the airline attendant can get into the restroom.

- Now that the airlines charge for blankets, pillows and food, you may need to provide the blanket, pillow and something to eat and drink. A small insulated lunch box will do the trick. Remember layers of clothing for warmth, planes are cool

- The airlines now charge for this extra-care service, so be prepared. Also, it is important that the person's dietary rules are followed.

- Be sure the airline understands that this person cannot be bumped, from the plane, or the gate changed. Multiple phone calls on your part may be necessary to make sure the traveling goes smoothly.

- Be sure the people who send your loved one home make the same arrangements in reverse.

- You may want to write everything down, including who you talked to at the airline, and provide this information to the person your loved one is visiting.

There will come a time when, even if the person with dementia says that they want to go on a trip, it is not really an option.

A friend of mine decided to take her mother to a family reunion for her aunt's 100th birthday. Due to meticulous planning, everything went very smoothly. My friend accompanied her mother. When they returned my friend reported that they had had a wonderful time, the only caveat being that her mother did not recognize a good many of the people there, got tired easily, and kept asking why they were there. Once they had been home for about a month, her mother had no memory of going to the reunion at all. My friend was just slightly disappointed she had made all the effort. Her intention was to give her mother a lasting memory of her family.

Chapter Thirty-six

PETS: BOB'S STORY

Bob moved into an apartment in our assisted living facility with Tessie, his cocker spaniel. Tessie's coat was caramel and white, and incredibly soft. The dog, for her part, was extremely friendly and loved everyone. In her world, no enemy existed. When she saw someone she knew coming down the hall, she would tug at her leash, jump, and yip in an effort to get the person's attention. Bob found this behavior incredibly appealing and smiled at her fondly, whenever she did it.

As time progressed, and getting around became more difficult, Bob found Tessie's outgoing greetings less endearing. It became harder for Bob to control the dog and still keep his balance. Bob took to leaving Tessie in his apartment more frequently and, of course, his leaving made Tessie all the more frantic to get out.

When the time came that Bob needed to use a walker to increase his stability, it was time for Tessie to go to live with Bob's daughter. Although he protested, it was obvious he was relieved to have Tessie go. Because Bob's daughter knew he would miss Tessie, she brought the animal to visit frequently. This worked out well, while Bob resided in his apartment. Tessie was one of those dogs that made everyone happy, and even the residents who were not "dog" people loved a visit from Tessie. Bob's daughter must have spent an extra hour whenever she visited Bob, just to allow everyone who wanted to, to pet and have time with Tessie.

Eventually Bob's dementia progressed even further, and his daughter wanted him moved to the increased care unit. All the caregivers on that unit, just loved Bob, as he still retained a sense of humor and never resisted care, which made him a delight to be around. Often he would talk about missing Tessie and would ask for her, forgetting he and his daughter had agreed to keep the dog with her family. When told about the arrangement, he readily accepted that Tessie would come to visit soon.

Near Christmas time, while shopping, one of the caregivers came across a mechanical dog that looked exactly like Tessie right down to her caramel and white coloring, but this one sported a red collar and leash. The plush dog would stand, sit, lie down and bark twice when the button was pushed. She gave the toy to Bob, who immediately fell in love with the it, and took to dragging it around by its leash while holding on to his walker. Sometimes he would even ask the caregivers to bring Tessie along when he ambulated from his room into the dining room where most activities took place. The stuffed Tessie would lie on the floor for hours while Bob was involved, ate a meal, or just talked to friends.

One day his daughter brought the real Tessie for a visit, and Bob basically ignored her. His daughter reminded him that Tessie was there to see him, at which point he lectured his daughter, "That's not Tessie. This is," he said, pointing to the stuffed animal lying quietly at his feet.

While this is a funny and charming story, it perfectly illustrates the point that individuals with dementia respond better when the things in their world are simple. They get confused and frightened when they must respond to changing stimulus. The adage, "keep it simple," really applies here.

Chapter Thirty-seven

DREAM STATE

One day, while sitting at my desk, there came a loud, frantic pounding at the office door. My first thought was that something was really wrong, but had it been a caregiver with serious news, she would have opened the door. When the pounding came a second time, I got up, crossed the room and opened the door. I was faced with a wild-eyed, breathless woman who demanded in a loud voice, "What did you do with my husband?"

I was so taken aback, I answered, "I didn't do anything."

She responded heatedly, "You must have taken him away! We were just making love, I turned over and he was gone. He wouldn't have just left me like that when we were making love!" Her distress was obvious and I was momentarily at a loss.

My assistant, who was privy to this onslaught, came to my rescue. "Oh, Marcia, your husband had to hurry to a meeting for his work, but he said he'd call and let you know when he would be back for you. I'm sorry, I thought he told you."

Marcia was only slightly mollified by this explanation, but left our office muttering and generally annoyed. The sadness of this story is that Marcia's husband had been dead for almost five years, and due to her dementia, she did not remember. Even though she had gone through the illness, death and services for him, she did not remember that he was gone. The good news was that she would not remember ten minutes later, either the dream about making love or the excuse my assistant gave about his going to a meeting. She would go on with her day as though none of this had happened.

This story illustrates another point regarding dementia. As people progress in this illness, they lose the ability to tell the difference between the dream and waking states. If someone dreams it, it happened. Thus, family members may hear stories that concern them, because what comes across is that their loved one is telling them something they believe to be true. We have all had the experience of having a particularly vivid dream. Sometimes this kind of dream, or at least the feelings it evokes, stays with us when we wake up and beyond. If the dream was unpleasant, we might get up, walk around, have a cup of tea or chocolate and even read to dispel the dream's feelings, but we always know it was a dream. Persons with dementia do not.

Unfortunately, this can also happen with television. Particularly if the person with dementia is still at home, monitoring their television watching is a must.

Gwen was a lady who moved into assisted living for memory care with a diagnosis of expressive aphasia brought on by a stroke. She knew what she wanted to say, but was embarrassed by her inability to express herself. She also had a diagnosis of MCI (Mild Cognitive Impairment). Gwen was a news "junkie" and had her television tuned to CNN, all day. Her son was an EMT, who worked varying shifts, so he would come to see her at different times.

As her dementia progressed she stayed in her room watching TV more and more. One night during a conflict in Iraq, an ambulance was blown up by terrorists and it was on the news. Gwen was inconsolable, screaming in the halls at two in the morning. When we finally figured out what had her so upset, we called her son to come in even though it was two-thirty in the morning, because she wouldn't believe his voice on the phone saying he was alive and unhurt. After all, she had seen it on television with her own eyes.

Psychologists tell us that our dreams are important and that having them helps us maintain our sanity. Unfortunately, the dream state does not do much for individuals with dementia, except momentarily confuse them. Hopefully they have only good dreams!

Chapter Thirty-eight

"I WANT TO GO HOME"...

I believe, without exception, that every person I have encountered with dementia has said the above phrase. Most family members have had the experience of hearing their loved one say it. Over time I have come to believe that these individuals are not asking to go to a particular place, but to return to a place in time where they felt safe and in control of their lives.

Remember when you were a child? For most of us, home represented a place of safety. A place we felt secure, knew we were loved, and knew we belonged. When dementia comes on, the people affected lose that feeling of knowing themselves.

The other phrase I hear frequently is "I feel so confused"—and they are confused. The individual knows something has changed, perhaps is wrong, and that their mind will not make sense of their surroundings.

I believe that individuals with dementia are like someone in a perpetual dream state. When one of us has a dream and wakes up, good or bad, we know instantly that we had a dream. For much of the time, people with dementia wander in a limbo state not knowing what exactly is real and desperately wanting to remember who they are and where they should be. What they do know is that they are not the same; they do not know what is wrong and they want to go back to where they were all right and in control. They want to go home.

If the person with dementia has had a positive relationship with their children, they will trust them most of all, but that does not mean the person will not say things that are hurtful or even incorrect and untruthful. Sometimes the person might a family member "the caregivers beat people when you aren't here." *Is that true?* the member will wonder. Yet, a check reveals no bruising on the loved one, and other residents are not afraid to ask for what they need, nor do they fear approaching a care giver. It is possible that the loved one's illusion was a memory from long ago; it is possible it was a dream? So if a loved says something unbelievable, a good response is, "Tell me more about that." Or, "Why do you think someone would do that?" Frequently, within the next couple of things they say, it will become clear where they got the idea.

The most important thing to do is meet them where they are. Do not deny their reality even if the tale is skewed, or bizarre. There was a gentleman who was very bright, a world-renowned businessman who had been Chairman of the Board for more than one international company. He had traveled the world extensively. One afternoon he brought a sheaf of papers to the tea table and, while all the other residents were having tea and cookies, he held forth about international finance and other important matters. He talked for about twenty minutes. He finished by announcing, "That is all I have to say," re-stacked his papers, and left the room. It clearly made him happy to talk to a group of people and he did this same routine for months. He had made his world into that which was familiar; he had gone home to the best of his ability.

The other compulsion this gentleman demonstrated was walking. He had severe kyphosis, a curving of the spine, so had to hold on to the hand rail that went around the room for support. The entire building had hand rails in every corridor, and around each public room, to aid the residents in ambulation. One day the Community Manager happened to come into the room, just as he started to walk. She asked him where he was going and he replied that he was going on the train across France. She asked if she could go along, at which point he took her arm and began walking, holding on to the hand rail with one hand and her with the other. He pointed out sights along the way, much to her delight. When they returned to the main room the CM told him that this was where she had to get off the train, said good-bye and thanked him for taking her along. He smiled, tipped an imaginary hat and continued on his way.

What could be more important than giving someone a "moment of joy?" All people with dementia have is what they are doing at the moment. They do not remember, and they have lost the capacity to anticipate. All there is, is *now*. When a loved one says something known to be untrue, the best approach is to find out more about what they are saying, and if necessary, offer sympathy for the situation.

One woman was convinced there was a conspiracy against her. She asked one of the male caregivers who he was, and at the same time told him there was this conspiracy. He replied that he was working with military intelligence in close cooperation with local law enforcement. When she objected that he did not know who was involved, he shared that they had arrested one conspirator and were building a case against another. This appeared to mollify her, but moments later she told him the conspirators were going to flog her, break her back, and poison her. He told her he would go to any lengths to protect her, and again she appeared to take in this information and feel better.

It is not always easy to hear the stories someone with Alzheimer's tells. Our first inclination, as it is with our children, is to bring them to reality and deny any potential harm. But unlike children, they cannot be brought into reality. Reassurance that they are safe, that you will take care of them, and not let any harm befall them is what they need most

Chapter Thirty-nine

KEEPING A LOVED ONE AT HOME

The generation that has or is getting dementia currently, has an inordinate fear of nursing homes, and who can blame them? Nursing homes, "back in their day" were grim places, one lady termed "ghettos for the elderly." Of course, this was before the move to patient-centered care, and predated special units for memory care. Today's nursing homes are not the places they once were, and are focused on rehabilitation rather than just warehousing the elderly. Some nursing homes do have permanent wings in which they care for people who cannot be kept at home, or need more care than can be provided by assisted living communities. There is not only a need, but a definite positive role nursing homes play, in the continuum of care.

Assisted living communities can be wonderful places and give older folks a place where they can interact with their peers. Believe it or not, this interaction is terribly important, as research appears to indicate that most individuals do better when they have this opportunity. Just like children need their peers, so do older folks. Who can talk about having children to someone who has not had them? Those people with different realities can sympathize, but they cannot empathize. In this same way, the elderly can talk to each other differently than they can with their children or younger people who have no frame of reference for what they are saying. The things they do can literally offend young people, like driving slowly, or talking about their illnesses. Perhaps some elders should not be driving, but their reaction time has slowed, and if they drive fast they are at greater risk. If they have no alternative, they drive, albeit slowly.

Just as young married couples talk about their kids, the elderly talk about their ailments, what the doctor said, and how a certain dinner made them feel.

If you think you should keep your parent with dementia at home with you, there are a number of things to keep in mind. Safety becomes paramount. Can this person get out of the house or yard? What steps can be ensure that the person will remain safe? In the early stages of dementia the person may be happy to stay put, near the house, or in the back yard. The problem is that, one day, they can just wander away. There is no way to tell when that day will come. Is your house child-proof, with locks on drawers and cabinets, and dangerous cleaning chemicals put away where they cannot be accessed? Are the throw rugs a danger? Does the person have difficulty walking? Will he or she use a walker? When you are not home, is there someone to stay with them? Are they safe alone? What about the kitchen, knives, microwave, etc.

Generally people are aware that a person with dementia cannot use the stove safely, but make the mistake of thinking that a microwave is safe. I cannot tell you how frequently I hear stories of individuals with dementia using a microwave inappropriately and starting fires.

I highly recommend that persons who are considering keeping their loved one at home look on the internet for Julie Winkour's *Sandwich Generation*, both for the information it provides and her personal experience, along with that of her husband Ed Kashi, and their children. Julie is a film producer who researched *Aging in America*, and felt she wanted to keep her father home when he was diagnosed with dementia. I agree with her, that the one-to-one care her dad received was special and positive for him. I do not agree that all communities lack one-to-one care. Smaller communities have the capacity to design their care to the needs of the individual, while at the same time providing someone with early dementia the companionship and activities they need. Julie also had a unique situation where both she and her husband could work at home much of the time as they did not have to go into an office. Still, Julie had management issues with the caregivers who came into her home. Anytime someone takes care of your loved one there will be issues, as no one can ever care for your loved one on the same level you do. But keep in mind that as dementia progresses, and although the person may need more physical care, they decline in awareness. They are not aware of the sacrifices anyone makes for them, you or a caregiver.

A community focusing on memory care can be a wonderful place where the caregivers give the residents not only the best physical care, but love them, and, like small children, the residents sense or feel that love. Near the end when someone with dementia may not even recognize their own family members, they feel safe with their caregivers, because they are familiar. I believe it is every person's responsibility to give their loved one the best care possible, to meet them where they are, and to give them as much good time as they can receive. Giving your life over to caring for someone with dementia is not necessary and can be detrimental to your relationship, both with them and with the others in your life. Their relationship to you, yours, to your significant other, and even your to your children can be affected. You need to ask what it is you believe, and what is the best answer for your family. You want to be there as a supportive son or daughter to your parent, but if you have to be the caregiver also, it may not be the most productive situation.

The other thing to consider is what kind of dementia your loved one has. Julie's dad only lived a couple of years after diagnosis; frequently people live much longer and their rate of decline is slower. Each family needs to decide what the best thing may be, given their financial situation and other factors which affect care. There is never an easy solution, and this kind of decision should be made with all family members, including the children.

Think long and hard about keeping a parent at home. This is not an easy decision to make. This is

not an easy disease to deal with under any
circumstances.

Chapter Forty

TOOLS THAT HELP

It is important to remember that dementia is different for everyone who has the disease. Not only are the symptoms different, but because each person is an individual, they can have exactly the same disease, and it will manifest itself with multiformity. As a primary person in someone's life, be as creative with memory aides as you want. If an idea works, keep it; if it does not, try something else, whether or not your loved one is in a dementia community.

Signs printed on white paper in block letters can help with a variety of facts. The obvious is labeling drawers: socks, underwear, sweaters, etc. or knives, forks and spoons (silverware). This does not mean that a person with dementia will remember what the items are used for, but they may. Issues like remembering to turn off the stove, or what one can put in a microwave safely may be obvious. For those, you might make a sign which says, USE ONLY WITH ANOTHER PERSON PRESENT.

Michelle S. Bourgeois is a speech pathology professor at Ohio State University. When she was doing her PhD research in the 1980s, she developed some of the first memory books, which use pictures and simple sentences to help people with memory problems.

Reading is a skill we learn over and over. That is to say, we learn to read beginning at age five or six (or earlier) and continue to learn, through this medium, for the rest of our lives. This skill, the act of reading, becomes part of our long term memory so it is less affected as dementia symptoms come on, which begin in the hippocampus with current memory.

Spoken words can confuse someone with dementia, but if they can read a simple sentence, they can understand better that which someone is trying to communicate. So, if you are riding in a car and your passenger repeatedly asks where you are going, answer them, but write down the answer on a pad and give the pad to that person.

One of the things that happens to people with dementia is they are going backward in time. Frequently they think of themselves as younger than they are. Sometimes they will not recognize themselves in a mirror. They may confuse their daughter with an aunt or sister who looks as that person used to look. They can think a son is actually an uncle or friend. One lady thought her son was her husband because they looked alike, and she saw herself as her son's age. Individuals may look for their children to come home from school, forget that they are retired, and expect to go to work or want to see a long deceased parent. Trying to reorient them at this juncture can be both confusing and painful, even if they believe you. The better approach is to go along with their reality for the present. For the moment, try distracting them. Later, you may give them a flash card which tells them who you are and reminds them, gently, who they are.

Behavior is another thing that can sometimes be helped by the use of flash cards. If a person is recalcitrant about, say, bathing or brushing their teeth a simple card which says SHOWERS MAKE ME FEEL GOOD, or MY MOUTH FEELS BETTER WHEN I BRUSH MY TEETH may work. These cards frequently will go a long way towards getting the person to cooperate.

Like young children, people with dementia develop their sixth sense and can tell if someone is patronizing them or does not really care about getting through to them. They will go along with you if they understand instinctively that their caregiver has their best interests at heart.

The use of labels and flash cards will not make a person's dementia better. It can help a loved one's caregiver have an easier time and be less frustrating for the individual. Try using any tool you can think of to evoke and help their memory. It will only work for a while, and then the disease will progress, and you may have to try something else.

Keep trying. It feels good to participate, and it does help. Resistance to care is not consistent, as individuals who have any form of dementia can go along with care one day and resist it the next. Flash cards can make a difference in both the dementia-disposed person's demeanor and their happiness.

A study done by Dr. Linda Buettner, who authored *Simple Pleasures*, shows the involvement of family members in a person's care can make a huge difference. Whether or not you put your loved one in a community that caters to dementia or you keep him or her at home, it is important to write a detailed history about that person. This history can give clues to the caregivers about how to get through and better communicate.

Chapter Forty-one

MASSAGE, AROMA, MUSIC, ART, EXERCISE, PET,

AND REMINISCENCE THERAPIES

I have addressed these therapies as a group because all are important and will help someone with most kinds of dementia. Obviously they will help some individuals more than others, depending on both individual preference and what diagnosis they have.

Massage Therapy will work for anyone who enjoys the feeling of being massaged, and it helps some individuals to relax. However, there are people who do not care to be touched, and forcing an experience on someone else—

especially someone with dementia—is always a bad idea. Massage should be gentle, with a goal of making the person feel good. Often this process can be accompanied by bathing and music, which can add to the entire experience. Massage can relieve minor pain and improve circulation. Sometimes chair massage is an acceptable alternative to having someone take off all their clothes, especially if the person is resistant. Massage is also an excellent way for a person to have human contact. When we are young we are frequently held by our parents, then by our spouse or significant other, but who holds an older person? Most of us need it and do not get it.

Aroma Therapy is not new. It has been used for thousands of years to ease stress and engender feelings of well-being. The ancients in Egypt used fragrant oils in the bath, to purify the air, and even repel insects. The essential oils of plants are now used in diffusers to stimulate appetite or relax individuals, and help them rest. There is some scientific evidence that essential oils, when used in diffusers, can positively affect people who have dementia. Individuals who have dementia operate on a gut level most of the time, unlike those of us who can think our way through a given problem. The difficulty with thinking is that we can block out what has the capacity to relax us.

Art Therapy can work on a lot of different levels of dementia. The tasks must be appropriate to the person's level of cognition, and the participants must be encouraged. Like little kids, people with dementia love to see their artwork displayed. Sometimes communities will have an Activities Director who facilitates these processes. For those at home, adult day care frequently provides this kind of activity. Whatever the discipline, art reaches out to everyone, and makes those who participate feel they are contributing.

Exercise is good for us. Even people in wheelchairs need to exercise. They can certainly lift their arms, and sometimes their legs or feet. Doing exercise, on a regular basis, keeps circulation moving and aids in strengthening older muscles. There are many classes in several venues that offer exercise if your loved one is still at home. Most assisted living communities offer exercise on a daily basis. Exercise helps with many issues, not the least of which are weight gain, heart health, and sleeping.

Reminiscence Therapy generally works best on individuals who are in Stages 3 to 5. Once a person stops speaking, it heralds a loss of function which includes historical memory and word retrieval. That does not mean, however, that individuals cannot benefit from story time, and they can frequently pay attention to the stories, even though they cannot participate. To listen to someone talk about the "old days" can make people with dementia feel part of the norm. Their historical memory lasts much longer than their current memory, and can aid in the person feeling a part of his or her generation.

Music has the ability to help everyone, regardless of their stage of dementia or level of health. Music is experienced in a different part of the brain from language and memory. Sometimes, people who are no longer able to utter speech are able to sing and remember the words to songs. I knew a lady who played the harmonica, and she played an entire song for me, the night before she died. I have seen music calm a person who was very upset at whatever was going on in his mind. A caregiver put on a classical piece of music for him and once he began to listen, he could sit down and forget his anger.

Most communities, and frequently adult day care facilities, will offer some sort of musical performance for the benefit of their charges. People who cannot sit still for five minutes, frequently have the ability to sit through an entire performance. Music reaches people as no other medium is able to do.

Currently, a degree in Music Therapy is available, and people with this degree are often called on to play for the dying. It has been my privilege to attend their playing and watch as the dying person was able to relax. It is an important thing to know what kind of music helps to sooth your loved one's personality, so that at the end, wherever they are, someone can put a disc on a player for them to aid them on their final journey.

Pet therapy can be a boon to any community. Anyone who has experienced the joy of unconditional love, and the relationship with an animal can reexperience this with a therapy dog. There are dogs specifically trained to not jump, to sit quietly, and be petted by anyone. Spending time with a pet can bring down blood pressure and engender a feeling of well-being. There are many pet therapists in every community that visit all the different facilities to give the residents the joy of having a pet without the responsibility. If your loved one is still at home, many of the therapy dogs can visit at a specific time. Therapy dogs visit hospitals, adult day care, nursing homes and various other facilities, regularly.

Chapter Forty-two

OCCUPATIONAL THERAPY AND ADULT DAY CARE

Occupational therapists (OT) are among the most helpful and creative people in health care. Their job is to help a person with or without dementia stay safe while preserving as much of their independence as possible. The OT can assess what skills the person still has and proceed to teach either the person or caregivers how to maximize these skills. They assist the person and the family in developing workable strategies for solving various problems in the environment. They look for ways to modify the bathroom, kitchen, and other living areas to reduce the risk of falls and dangerous accidents, as well as generally safety-proofing the area in which the person lives.

When the person with dementia progresses, or when problems with coordination, dressing and bathing arise, OTs will be able to recommend different kinds of solutions. OTs can also help with obtaining specialty equipment like raised toilet seats, wheelchairs, walkers, etc. The physician will write an order following the OTs recommendation.

OTs can be located through a physician, nursing service, or in the phone book under "physical therapy." They are licensed, so they must meet certain standards.

Adult day care centers provide socialization and structure for people who have early to moderate dementia. Their programs are, for the most part, activity-based; they focus on keeping a person with dementia engaged, and using the skills they still have. They often offer movement, exercise, listening to music, crafts, and singing. Frequently centers are open seven days per week, and people can enroll their loved ones for half or full-day sessions. Meals are typically included. If the daycare is not affordable, talk to the people at the agency; sometimes partial or full scholarships are available for those in need. Also, the local Alzheimer's Association may assistance or offer referrals to others who provide services. Daycare may also be covered by Long-Term Care Insurance. Medicare will not pay for it, but in some states, Medicaid will.

You may find your loved one resistant to daycare, but keep trying to work it into a routine. Like children when they go to kindergarten, they may resist at first, but may really like it once they get there. The people who run adult day care know what they are doing, and are used to dealing with people who have dementia. They will also be able to tell you when your loved one is no longer appropriate for their program.

Chapter Forty-three

SURGERY

The only justification for doing surgery on people with dementia is to alleviate pain. As with children, pain for a person with dementia is total. There is no way to mitigate it by explanation or distraction. Persons with dementia are not able to ameliorate pain as adults can by the knowledge that the pain is temporary or that it can be medicated.

All surgery is not the same, and sometimes what is required of the patient after the surgery a person with dementia is incapable of doing. Cataract surgery is no big deal for a cognitively intact adult, but for a person with dementia, it becomes next to impossible. Someone with dementia cannot keep their hands off the operative eye because it itches. One can tell them over and over, but they do not remember what you have said.

There was a particular woman whose mother, Beth, needed cataract surgery. Beth was normally very compliant, especially when her daughter told her to do something. The daughter planned to stay overnight, on a cot, in Beth's apartment, in order to ensure her cooperation. The daughter's precautions did not protect her mother's eye. Beth removed the patch during the night and rubbed her eye, displacing the new lens. Beth ended up not being able to see well out of the operative eye. Her daughter felt guilty because she was sure Beth was capable of following the doctor's instructions with her help. Needless to say, the daughter did not have the cataract taken off the other eye.

The only reason surgery is valid is to end pain, if there is simply no alternative. A hot gall bladder or a broken hip will not fix themselves. If a person with dementia must have surgery, steps should be taken to have the patient attended twenty-four hours a day, seven days per week, until whatever needs to heal, does heal.

What is the outcome if the person with dementia has surgery? What is the result if this person goes without surgery? Will their suffering increase? Talk to the physician, and perhaps Hospice, before making your decision. Be sure that all family members understand what is happening, and are willing to go along with a particular decision.

Chapter Forty-four

THEORY OF PERSONALITY

When we are children, we learn from our parents, teachers and peers what is acceptable in terms of our behavior. Over time, we take on a social veneer, which is the political glue that allows us to function as a member of society. For instance, if we tell our boss what a jerk he is, we will probably get fired. Telling him is a no-no. However, as dementia increases the essential personality of the individual evidences itself.. That is to say, the social veneer we have spent a life time accruing begins to disappear. So, if a person is negative or mean-spirited underneath, basic traits reveal themselves. Conversely, if a person is basically a happy soul, that also evidences itself.

Many family members have told me how embarrassed they were when, at a restaurant, their loved one remarked on the fat woman sitting next to them, or stared at the man with one arm. As children, we learn that these observations must be kept to oneself; with dementia, all stops are off.

It is important to understand that more than just being embarrassed, a part of their brain quits functioning and, like precognitive children, they actually do not understand that they are being rude. They may in fact be trying to understand what they are seeing.

Individuals with dementia can become paranoid about things that are meaningless or they can become an unmitigated delight. Freed from the rules of society, they can love and be loved without reserve. They can relish love as they may have never been able to do when they were more aware.

It is interesting to note that family members are rarely surprised when someone is angry or nasty. When questioned, they recall multiple times when their loved one's reactions to events were difficult or the person refused to cope. Individuals who have spent a life time manipulating others with their behavior get more manipulative when they have dementia, not less.

Closet alcoholism in individuals you would not suspect can surface, and if family members have their own issues, they may deny that there is a problem.

Sometimes family members are surprised at how lovely, warm, and sweet their person with dementia can act. If you ask them, they will frequently remember the person being shy, or kept down by the presence of a dominating spouse. Perhaps, to keep peace, the person functioned in a particular way, but now, with dementia, they can be themselves. This can make the time they have with their parent bittersweet because they know the time is finite and yet they have found this wonderful parent they did not know existed. They are frequently grateful for every day with this person.

Is there anything that can be done for a cranky individual? Usually this person's primary care physician can prescribe a mild mood elevator, which in some cases helps, but it is not always an answer. If the person is an unhappy person, then that is who they are. What this knowledge does is help both the family and the caregiver to not take personally what this person says or does.

Of course, there are individuals who become violent, and unfortunately they must be medicated so that they do not hurt themselves or anyone else. These are the saddest cases because it is almost impossible to give this kind of person any moments of joy.

Chapter Forty-five

TAKE CARE OF YOURSELF

The single hardest thing to do is accept the fact that someone you love has the disease of dementia. *Dementia* is a blanket term covering all degenerative brain disorders. While some forms of dementia have specific symptoms, all dementias are progressive, and eventually render the person with the disease into a state where they require help with activities of daily living.

No one is capable of taking care of a person with dementia alone. It is not a one-person job, even if you are a professional. You must have aid. Help can take many forms and there are a lot of resources available. (See the appendix for a list of web sites and books to read, and be sure to call your local chapter of the Alzheimer's Society, or the Council on Aging, for starters.)

Even if you have limited funds, you can get help. Be sure to check with Medicare and Medicaid to see what services your loved one may be qualified to receive once diagnosed with dementia.

Get yourself to a support group, even if you are not a "touchy feely" type of person. There is a good deal of information and practical help that can be found in a support group. For one thing, no one understands what you are dealing with like someone else who is going through the same thing. Your friends may sympathize, but group members can empathize.

Educate yourself. Read, search the internet, and generally learn all you can about whatever form of dementia you loved one has. Research will allow you to make a more informed and appropriate set of decisions. Bring your family members along. They need help to support you and your loved one emotionally. They need to be on the same page as you are. The result of family unification is that you and they are able to obtain the best help for your loved one and his/her particular type of dementia.

Taking care of yourself may feel like you are being selfish, but consider that if you do not take care of yourself you will not have the energy necessary to take care of your loved one. Guilt is a wasted emotion. It gets you absolutely nowhere. Let go of it and put your energies into something productive.

Going to a meeting, putting your loved one in a community that offers respite care, having help come in a couple of days a week; whatever form taking care of yourself requires, do it. You need to have some kind of life and do those things you need to do for yourself. Remember, this disease will eat you up, if all you do is take care of a loved one with dementia. Learn what your limits are and refuse when asked to go beyond those limits.

I realize that in the beginning the person with dementia appears capable and you want them to do as much as they can, in order to maintain their independence. The difficulty comes when they surprise you and do the unexpected. There is no way to expect specific changes, but stay on the alert for general changes in behavior. Keep close contact with your loved one's physician, and keep him updated on the changes you are seeing—for instance, wandering at night. You must get your rest, even if the person with dementia changes their diurnal rhythms. Remember, they can nap during the day; you probably cannot.

Taking care of yourself, while you are taking care of someone with dementia can definitely be a challenge. Do not try to do alone. The life you save may be your own.

Chapter Forty-six

WHAT TO BRING ALONG

As a family or on your own, if you have decided to move your loved one into a community, there are items you want to bring with you. Additionally, there are items your loved one does not need, and as their dementia progresses, can even become hazardous.

In my tenure as head nurse, I have had to remove, scissors, knives, nail clippers, screw drivers, needles, pins, cleaning chemicals, and a plethora of other items from a resident's room that were dangerous because the person no longer used these items appropriately. Like little children, their thinking can be tangential. Any sharp item can be dangerous in the hands of someone with dementia.

One gentleman used a large pair of nail clippers to remove the baseboard in his room. He said he was sure "they were hiding things behind the baseboard." He only did this in the late afternoon, and would then complain the next morning that the baseboards in his room were coming apart. We were initially unaware that he even had the nail clippers.

Your loved one does not need anything sharp, including push pins or tacks. All the things they could need temporarily—like a hammer or nails—can usually be provided by the community or a family member, and taken away after they are used.

Following is a list of items that you do want to bring:

Continence pads or pull-ups

Pads for the bed and a plastic mattress cover

Non-toxic soap

Baby shampoo

Non-toxic or edible hand/skin lotion

Paper and pencils/pens

Tooth paste and toothbrush

Floss

Hair brush

Comfortable clothing in outfits

Shoes with non-skid soles

Slippers that stay on someone's feet (not skuffies)

Comfortable bras (or sports bras) for women

T-shirts for men

Underwear (do not bring if person is wearing pull-ups)

Cotton socks

Ted hose, if used. These should be put on in the morning and taken off in the evening, be hand rinsed, and hung on the towel rack to dry. Putting Ted Hose in a dryer will make the elastic warp and become ineffective, thus more than one pair should be provided. You may want to check with your loved one's primary care physician or cardiologist to be sure that TED hose are still necessary. Individuals with dementia arrive at a point where they do not care about swollen ankles. They feel that Ted hose are too tight.

If there are other items you feel your loved one will simply not do without, bring them along, but advise the management; you can always remove the items later, once your loved one forgets about them.

Check occasionally to see if your loved one still feels they need that item, like panty hose.

Over-the-counter items like Tums, hemorrhoid creams, pads, or Tylenol are drugs. Most people do not think of them as such, reserving that designation for prescription drugs. Even vitamins or nutritional supplements require a doctor's order when a person is going into an assisted living facility. The problem arises when a person with dementia forgets they have taken something, and takes another. Many over-the-counter drugs have limits on how and when their drug should be taken. For instance, Tylenol taken too often can be toxic to the liver. All drugs should be surrendered to the nursing staff and doled out to the residents according to the doctor's prescription. The benefit is that if someone has a headache and asks for pain medication, a record is kept of the dose they received. Sometimes a resident will not get relief and ask for medication a second time. The nurse giving out the drugs can then alert the family and physician that the over-the-counter medication is not effective or requires different dosing.

Alcohol is a drug. A legal drug, but a drug none the less, and it may have interactions with other drugs being taken. Alcohol is contraindicated anytime someone is receiving an anti-psychotic drug or even some antibiotics. Go over your loved one's list of medications with their physician to be certain there are no contraindications on the list. Sometimes a physician will say that giving a person with dementia an occasional drink is all right, but you need to monitor it because a person with dementia has no intellectual stops. Either the person does not remember that he or she had a drink or they want another because it feels good. The same is true even of candy.

One woman kept bringing her uncle bags of candy for his room. She said she wanted him to have something to snack on. Apparently he had always been a big candy eater and she did not want to deprive him during his last days. The problem was, he could not remember how much candy he had eaten and would refuse to eat some meals because he felt full..

No one's disease remains static. Frequently families will put a loved one into a community and fail to recognize that the person's disease will continue to progress. Progression does not stop because the person is receiving professional care.

Chapter Forty-seven

WHEN IS A NURSING HOME APPROPRIATE?

A nursing home is appropriate when the person with dementia needs those services only a nursing home can provide. For instance, if someone cannot walk, is too heavy, and cannot make a successful transfer from bed to chair, chair to bath bench, or bath bench to wheelchair, it is time to research nursing homes.

Sometimes a dementia resident will need a nursing home for rehabilitation, for instance, if they break an ankle or a hip in a fall. Individuals may go to a nursing home immediately after the acute care phase of a hospital. After a short period, they may be returned to either assisted living or their home, just as soon as physical therapy thinks the person has reached his or her plateau. That is, the individual has progressed as far as therapy expects them to go. Physical therapy representatives may even recommend that the person go back to their place of residence, with the addition of home physical therapy, particularly if the person with dementia needs the routine of their community to support them emotionally.

Dementia progresses slowly, and physical deterioration happens slowly, so for the most part, families have plenty of time to figure things out and pick the place that best meets the needs of their loved one. Some nursing homes are not suited to a dementia resident who can walk or get around independently. Someone who is wheelchair bound and requires a three-person transfer may only be able to go to a nursing home. Sometimes concomitant health issues make a nursing home a better solution than assisted living.

Most assisted living facilities are not allowed to take care of a person who has a stage three (or higher) decubitus ulcer. This situation would require a nursing home because the person would require twenty-four hour nursing care. It should be noted that decubitus ulcers are measured by stages, where stasis ulcers (from inadequate blood perfusion) are not. Decubitus ulcers may be taken care of under the direction of a physician until they reach stage three. Stasis ulcers are either healing or non-healing, and should be attended by either a wound clinic or a wound nurse along with an attending physician.

In general, the people who make up the current older generation have an inordinate fear of nursing homes, because they either had a parent who had a bad experience in one, or have had a family member who died in one. They equate all nursing homes and assisted living with death, or warehousing of the elderly, and do not want to go there at any cost. They will attempt to extract a promise from their children, to "never send me to such a place." Frequently they are dealing with a predetermined fear and not reality.

If a family member has the appropriate finances, physical-care setup, and wants to keep a loved one at their home, it is always an option. However, it should be noted that most research shows that the elderly, with or without dementia, need peers just as we all do. Socialization is a crucial part of who we are. Of course, there are exceptions. As in every endeavor, no one mold fits all.

Chapter Forty-eight

DEATH

For people from our American culture, there is no subject harder to discuss than death. It is becoming slightly easier now that the population has aged, and more people are turning to Hospice. Death really needs to be discussed though, or people can die alone and frightened because the people who support them are too fearful to address death as a subject. Though the death experience is always painful, it does not have to always be dreadful. Mostly, people going through the experience need support. Family is important, but professionals can help a great deal.

In 1978, when my father was dying of gall stones blocking the bile duct (a condition that is not normally a terminal one), my sister and I came together at a Florida Critical Care unit and were completely dumbfounded about what to do. One of Dad's nurses whispered to me, "Ask for a death and dying counselor." She had to whisper it to me because in those days nurses were not allowed to tell families what was available to them. We asked for one, and the information she gave us allowed us to make good decisions and ask the appropriate questions of the physician. More importantly, it enabled us to act as a single personality, both in caring for my father and when it came to the end, allowing him to die with peace and dignity.

Though most people would opt not to die if they could, it is a truth that no one gets out of this life alive. Rich or poor, capable or mentally handicapped, everyone dies. Most of us have heard about the person who dies of a sudden heart attack, and most of us would sign up for that kind of easy death. What people really do not want to do is suffer. Moreover, we feel badly when a friend dies of some kind of slow cancer, because we know suffering is involved, not just by the person doing the dying, but also by the family.

Talking about the person's deepest wishes, acknowledging their pain (physical as well as psychic), giving them emotional support, and even a break to help them find their balance, are all crucial pieces in the process. Compassion for the person doing the dying is critical for both the person and the family members. One needs to be around others who loved that person as well. Nothing is harder than mourning alone.

In some ways it is harder to have a person with dementia die. Frequently there are things left unsaid because someone with dementia does not understand. There are occasions when family members are so fearful of pain medication that they want to withhold it, in the hope that their loved one will be aware at the end. Someone with dementia is not going to wake up and give them a last blessing. If a person has dementia, withholding pain medication will only increase their suffering. They do not know what is happening to them or why. To some degree this is a blessing, because they know neither fear nor depression.

The family, on the other hand, is not spared. If there was a problem, if things were left unsaid, it is too late to remedy that situation now. There are, however, things that can be done. The family can make a conscious effort to come together. They can talk about their relationships with the dying person, their history and whatever they experienced with that person. Frequently getting another view of an event can be a healing experience. It can free us of perceived and unnecessary guilt. *Guilt is a wasted emotion!* A sibling's story can make clear a parent's behavior that was previously thought to be one way and was really another. This is the greatest recommendation for keeping one's life relationships current.

One of my patients, Hank, who did not take many medications, and was seen by his primary care physician regularly, lived in an adult assisted living community. Though he was suffering some memory loss, it was minor, and he was generally enjoying his life.

One Friday he was in particularly fine spirits, as both his daughters were coming to visit the following weekend. As in most adult communities, the noon meal is the largest, giving slow stomachs a chance to digest their intake. After eating a hearty meal, he played cards for a couple of hours with three friends. Around 2:20 or so, he told the group he was a little tired and headed to his room for a nap. He took the elevator to the second floor, walked down the hall toward his room, when he got to the corner, he fell to the floor dead.

One of the caregivers saw him and called nursing on her radio immediately. By the time I reached him, in less than a minute, he was no longer breathing. I listened to his heart with my stethoscope and heard his heart flutter, then stop. I listened for a full minute but no other sound or beat occurred. Even though I knew he had a "Do Not Resuscitate Order," I had to call 911 because his body needed to be moved from the hall floor to his bedroom.

I began calling his daughter who lived within a couple of hours drive, but was unsuccessful in reaching her. I even tried reaching the daughter who lived in California but to no avail, and I did not want to leave a message under the circumstances. I continued trying to call his local daughter every hour on the hour all through the night, but was not successful in reaching her until the next afternoon. She told me that she had gone for an overnight sail with her sister and had been incommunicado for about nineteen hours.

The family had previously made all the final arrangements, so I was able to notify the funeral home, and they came to pick up the body.

When his daughters finally got to our community, we spent time crying together because we would miss him; he was such a good man. His eldest daughter said something that day that I will remember always. She said, "My father did for me the last great favor he could do. He did not make me watch him suffer."

It is my recommendation that you talk to your parents about what they want done when they die, both as to ceremony and disposal, before they become ill. Do they favor burial, cremation, or donation to science, etc.? If they make decisions about what they want, others don't have to.

Chapter Forty-nine

In Closing

LIVING WITH DEMENTIA

The best anyone can do is offer general guidelines to make the process of going through this illness slightly less painful. The general guidelines I offer come from years of working with families to make the transition a little smoother and easier for everyone involved.

Unfortunately, there will always be individuals who, because of their own issues, cannot take into consideration what is best for a loved one. There are some rules that can help, and foremost among these is checking with your loved one's physician. The others follow suit: get your loved one diagnosed; talk to family members so that the best possible solution for your loved one can be found—like the decision to keep the person at home or place them in a facility. Treat yourself well, and let go of guilt. Get the advice of an Elder Attorney. And remember that this part of life isn't all there is to life, so seek to provide yourself and your loved one with moments of joy!

About the Author

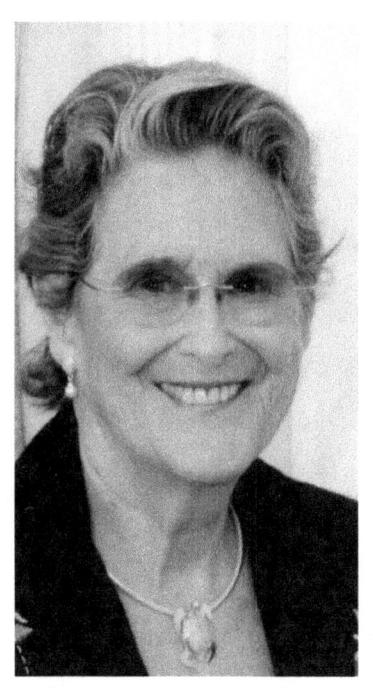

Melinda Fengel, RN, BSN, received her Bachelor's Degree in Nursing from the Leinhard School of Nursing, part of Pace University in New York. She has held licenses to practice in both Arizona and Washington. Melinda's varied career has included positions in personnel, law enforcement, and nursing. She lives with her husband of thirty-three years in Prescott Valley, Arizona.

Appendix A

BOOKS AND DISCS

BOOKS

No More Words, by Reeve Lindberg - ISBN:0-7432-0313-5

The Everything Health Guide to Alzheimer's Disease, by Maureen Dezell with Carrie Hill, PhD.-ISBN 10:1-60550-124-7

The Alzheimer's Answer Book, by Charles Atkins, M.D. – Sourcebooks, Inc.

On Death and Dying, Elizabeth Kubler-Ross – ISBN 0-02-089130-X

How We Die, Reflections on Life's Final Chapter, by Sherwin B. Nuland, M.D. – ISBN 0-679-41461-4.

Melinda Fengel, RN, BSN

Creating Moments of Joy for the Person with Alzheimer's or Dementia, by Jolene Brackey

Diagnosis and Management of Alzheimer's Disease and Other Dementias, by Robert C. Green, MD, MPH – ISBN 1-884735-97-7

DISCS

ACCPETING THE CHALLENGE, Produced by the Alzheimer's Association of Eastern North Carolina, starring Teepa Snow. www.alznc.org/bookstore.htm

There is a Bridge, Produced by Memory Bridge, Chicago IL, www.memorybridge.or

This list is, by no means, a full list of available books on the subject, but they are they are among my favorites. These books give good information which is what so many people need when faced with this devastating illness.

Appendix B

LIST OF WEB SITES

http://www.alzforum.org/new/detail

http://www.alz.org

http://www.alzheimers.org

ADEAR (Alzheimer's Disease Education and Referral Center)

> (800-438-4380 a service of the National Institute on Aging (NIA)

http://www.tangledneuron.info (a layperson reports on memory loss, Alzheimer's & dementia

http://www.facebook.com/pages/Teepa-Snow/94951408338

http://www.johnshopkinshealthalerts.com

http://www.alzheimersanddementia.org

http://www.neuroassist.com/dementia.htm

http://www.peoplespharmacy.com

http://cdr.rfmh.org

http://www.ninds.nih.gov

http://www.nihseniorhealth.gov

http://www.alzfdn.org

http://www.eldercare.gov

http://www.caregiver.org

http://www.aricept.com

http://www.mayoclinic.com

http://www.aafp.org/afp

http://www.namenda.com

http://www.exelonpatch.com

http://www.neuroassist.com

http://www.emedicinehelth.com

http://www.cdc.gov

http://www.medicinenet.com

http://www.aging-parents-and-elder-care.com

http://www.ask.com

http://www.natural-living-for-women.com

http://www.FTD-Picks.org

http://www.PolyMem.com

http://www.almosthomedoc.org